Unraveling AIDS

The Independent Science and Promising Alternative Therapies

Mae-Wan Ho, Ph.D., Sam Burcher, Rhea Gala, Veljko Veljković, Ph.D.

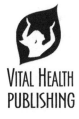

VITAL HEALTH
PUBLISHING

Unraveling AIDS

Published in 2005 by Vital Health Publishing, Ridgefield, CT

Cover Design: On the Dot Designs
Cover Photo by Adrian Dreamweaver, Dreams of Fire, South Africa
Interior Book Design: Cathy Lombardi

Published by: Vital Health Publishing
               P.O. Box 152
               Ridgefield, CT 06877
               Office phone: 203-794-1009; Orders: 877-VIT-BOOKS
               Web site: www.vitalhealthbooks.com
               E-mail: info@vitalhealthbooks.com

Disclaimer
Serious diseases should always be treated under medical supervision.
Never delay in seeking medical advice if you have any persisting medical
or psychological condition. The material in this book is for educational
purposes only and is not intended for use in diagnosing or treating
any individual.

Printed in the United States of America

ISBN: 1-890612-47-2
Library of Congress Control Number: 2005931281

Vital Health Publishing is committed to the goals of the Green Press Initiative
and to preserving Endangered Forests and conserving natural resources.
This book is printed on 30% postconsumer recycled paper.

Contents

Preface

AIDS (acquired immune deficiency syndrome) was identified as a global pandemic and "a threat to world security" by the Clinton administration in July 2000. President George W. Bush has pledged $15 billion to combat AIDS, and additional hundreds of millions of dollars have been donated by rich countries and charitable foundations.

Yet every aspect of the disease has been subject to acrimonious debate. Is AIDS a real disease? Is it a single disease? What is the real extent of the AIDS pandemic? Does HIV (Human Immunodeficiency Virus) cause AIDS? Is AIDS sexually transmitted? Do conventional anti-HIV drugs do more harm than good? Are the candidate anti-HIV vaccines effective, or even safe? Are there safe and effective treatments that can be made widely available at affordable costs?

Why does AIDS attract so much controversy? Part of the answer is that big pharmaceutical companies profit from the sale of lucrative drugs and hope to profit even more from effective AIDS vaccines, which are still in the pipelines after more than two decades. AIDS is perhaps the most-researched yet most-misunderstood disease in the world, about which the most misinformation is spread for political purposes.

Consequently, the multibillion-dollar international projects for addressing the "AIDS pandemic" may well miss their targets of alleviating suffering and death, and could even make things worse.

Our motivation in producing this book was to unravel the complex scientific debates surrounding the AIDS pandemic and to review treatments that are safe, effective, and affordable by all. We believe a great deal can be done to alleviate human suffering without turning AIDS into a political football.

This book goes to press amid news of a major scandal that has triggered a congressional hearing. U.S. government-funded researchers in top research institutions have been testing toxic AIDS drugs on hundreds of the most vulnerable orphaned and foster children over the past two decades, often without the legal protections for the children required in some states, exposing these children to the risks of research and serious side effects. It is all the more important that the information presented in this book become widely available to prevent further such abuses of basic human rights.

Mae-Wan Ho

Authorship and Acknowledgments

Dr. Mae-Wan Ho has written Chapters 1, 2, 3, 5, 6, 7, 9, 10, 12, 13, 15, 16, and 25; Sam Burcher has written Chapters 4, 14, 17, 19, 20, 21, and 22; Rhea Gala has written Chapters 8, 11, and 18; and Dr. Veljko Veljković has written Chapter 24. Burcher and Ho have jointly written Chapter 23. Dr. Ho is general editor for the volume. Dr. Veljković has commented on many chapters and has greatly influenced the contents.

Earlier versions of Chapters 3, 4, 8, 9, 10, 14, 17, 20, and 23 have appeared in successive issues of the quarterly magazine *Science in Society*, published by the Institute of Science in Society (www.i-sis.org.uk), and Chapters 3, 4, 14, 20, and 23 have appeared in *AIDS: In Search of a Social Solution*, published by Third World Network and People's Health Movement, Penang, Malaysia, 2004.

We thank Dr. David Rasnick (University of California, Berkeley); Dr. Howard Urnovitz (Chronix Biomedical); Dr. Aldar Bourinbaiar and Dr. Vichai Jirathitikal (Immunitor); Dr. Nigel Gericke, Dr. Carl Albrecht, and Professor Ben-Erik van Wyk (PhytoNova); Professor Harold Foster (University of Victoria); and John James (*AIDS Treatment News*) for answering numerous questions about their work and commenting on drafts of some of the chapters.

Dr. Joe Cummins played a crucial role in keeping us abreast of the relevant scientific literature. Our other colleagues in the Institute of Science in Society, Lim Li Ching, Andy Watton, and Julian Haffegee, provided essential moral and physical support that made our work possible. Bili Goldberg's e-mail list kept us in touch with much of relevant literature on HIV/AIDS over the years.

We wish to express our deep appreciation to our publisher, David Richard of Vital Health Publishing, for inspiring and encouraging us to greatly improve an earlier version of this manuscript.

We are grateful to the Denis Guichard Foundation for a grant toward producing this work, and to Third World Network for major support.

Statement of the Publisher and Authors

The publisher and the authors wish to express their thanks for all of the independent research that has made this book possible.

We offer the information contained herein in the spirit of open scientific inquiry into the causes of the AIDS disease and the most effective means of preventing and treating it. None of the theories, research studies, or treatment protocols discussed in this book are definitive. In fact, there remain more open-ended questions about HIV and AIDS, in terms of causality, diagnosis, prevention, and treatment, than there appear to be solid answers.

These questions, however, are of themselves critically important and should not be overlooked in the rush to find a medical solution to the AIDS pandemic. The publisher and the authors agree that the primary purpose and value of this book is not in the questions it answers but in the questions it raises. Our hope is that the perspectives presented herein will contribute favorably to the scientific dialogue about AIDS by criticizing orthodox theories and solutions and highlighting the most promising alternative theories and therapies. We place this information in the public forum trusting that its value will be tested and proven on the whole, if not in every particular.

The publisher and the authors wish to emphasize that this book is a work of scientific inquiry, not of practicing medicine. We do not personally or professionally endorse or censure any of the tests, drugs, nutrients, or treatments of the AIDS disease or of HIV. Nor do we personally or professionally endorse or censure any individual, organization, or government currently or previously involved in AIDS research, diagnosis, or treatment. Most importantly, we do not advise or condone *unprotected* sex in relationship to transmission of HIV or the AIDS disease. In our opinion, the use of a medically approved condom during sex is an advisable and necessary precaution for AIDS prevention at this time.

AIDS: A Global Pandemic

FRIGHTENING FIGURES ON THE AIDS PANDEMIC MAKE HEADLINES
ALL OVER THE WORLD. BUT DO THE FIGURES CONCEAL
THE REAL CAUSES OF HUMAN SUFFERING?

LATEST ESTIMATES

Figures from the Joint United Nations Program on AIDS (see box) released at the end of December 2003 claim 40 million affected with HIV or AIDS worldwide,[1] and within the year, 3 million people have died while 5 million new cases were recorded, the vast majority in sub-Saharan Africa. AIDS is also reported to be fast becoming a major problem in China, India, and Russia.

These horrendous figures of the "global AIDS pandemic" are widely reported, not only in newspapers and popular magazines, but also in scientific journals.[2]

Yet practically every aspect of the global AIDS pandemic has been challenged, from the reality of AIDS disease to the effectiveness and safety of expensive treatments with conventional pharmaceutical drugs. Big money is involved, which invariably clouds the picture.

For example, in July 2004, the Joint United Nations Program on AIDS (UNAIDS) figures were revised downward: 38 million were reported to be carrying the virus worldwide (2 million fewer than at the end of 2003), and the figure for sub-Saharan Africa was cut by 1.6 million to 25 million, while only 2.2 million died of AIDS, compared to 3 million in 2003.[3]

South Africa's figures have shrunk by 33 percent, according to the findings of the Actuarial Association of South Africa for 2002: about 5 million, instead of the earlier projected 7.5 million based on findings for 2000.[4]

HIV/AIDS Worldwide

At the end of 2003, an estimated 40 million people worldwide—37 million adults and 2.5 million children younger than fifteen years—are living with HIV/AIDS. Approximately two thirds (26.6 million) live in sub-Saharan Africa; another 18 percent (7.4 million) live in Asia and the Pacific.

Worldwide, approximately 11 in every 1,000 adults aged fifteen to forty-nine are infected with HIV. In sub-Saharan Africa, about 8 percent of all adults in this age group are HIV infected.

An estimated 5 million new HIV infections occurred worldwide during 2003; that is about 14,000 infections each day. More than 95 percent of these new infections occurred in developing countries, and nearly 50 percent were among females.

In 2003, approximately 2,000 children under the age of fifteen years and 6,000 young people aged fifteen to twenty-four years became infected with HIV every day.

In 2003 alone, HIV/AIDS-associated illnesses caused the deaths of approximately 3 million people worldwide, including an estimated half a million children younger than fifteen years.

Source: Joint United Nations Program on AIDS

EXTRAVAGANT PLEDGES

On December 1, 2003, World AIDS Day, the World Health Organization (WHO) and UNAIDS in Geneva unveiled their "three-by-five" plan to provide anti-HIV drugs to 3 million people in developing countries by 2005.[5] This represents only about half the people worldwide most in need of treatment and will cost $5.5 billion.

In his 2003 State of the Union address, President George W. Bush pledged a total of $15 billion over five years to fight HIV/AIDS in developing countries, especially in Africa.[6,7] Unfortunately, only $2 billion of the first year's expected $3 billion was made available, and funding appeared to be tied to the countries' purchase of conventional pharmaceutical drugs and their acceptance of genetically engineered crops. The allocated budget for 2005 is even less generous. The White House has requested only

$2.8 billion for programs to fight HIV/AIDS, tuberculosis, and malaria globally, with just a portion of this money going to Africa.

In India, where more people are said to be infected with HIV than any country except South Africa, Health Minister Sushma Swaraj said the government was in negotiations with Indian drug companies to get "rock-bottom drug prices" for AIDS patients. Indian patients could receive a commonly used triple-drug regimen for less than 20 cents a day, compared to the current cost of at least $1 a day, an industry source said.

Across the rest of Asia, in China, Japan and Thailand, celebrities are lending their glitter to the fight against AIDS and the arrival of big bucks. Spending on AIDS rose 50 percent, from $3.1 billion in 2002 to $4.7 billion in 2003, although it was still only half of what was needed, according to Peter Piot, UNAIDS' executive director.

In the chapters following, we shall look into the real extent of the AIDS epidemic; some of the main controversies surrounding the diagnosis and causes of the disease; the efficacy and safety of AIDS vaccines; and the side effects of expensive conventional anti-HIV drugs in contrast to some safe and effective treatments that can be made widely available at affordable costs.

What Is AIDS Disease?

NUMEROUS QUESTIONS REMAIN OVER THE DIAGNOSIS OF AIDS.

AIDS DIAGNOSIS IS A MATTER OF DEFINITION

By definition, AIDS can leave one vulnerable to all kinds of "opportunistic" infections that take advantage of weakened immune defenses, but detection of antibodies to HIV in the patient's blood defines whether someone has AIDS, as decreed by the U.S. Centers for Disease Control and Prevention's Revised Classification System for HIV Infection and Expanded Surveillance Case Definitions for AIDS published in 1993.[1]

So the detection of anti-HIV antibodies in someone with diarrhea, dementia, Kaposi's sarcoma (a form of cancer), cervical cancer, pneumonia, tuberculosis, and so on would yield a diagnosis of AIDS, whereas another person with exactly the same symptoms who does not have anti-HIV antibodies would be classified as free of AIDS. That's how it is in the United States and Europe.

But AIDS in Africa is something else. It is almost always diagnosed without testing for HIV, because the tests are too costly. American public health officials established a different definition of AIDS in Africa at a conference held in October 1985 in Bangui, Central African Republic. The Bangui definition allows health professionals to diagnose AIDS in Africa based only on the symptoms and signs.

These symptoms and signs are not new. According to Dr. David Rasnick of the University of California at Berkeley, a prominent AIDS dissident, or critic of the prevailing view of HIV/AIDS, they "represent the same old diseases and conditions that have plagued Africans for countless generations before AIDS."[2] So, for example, tuberculosis, fever, diarrhea, wasting, and other diseases of poverty have now been reclassified as AIDS.

UNRELIABLE METHODS FOR DETECTING HIV ANTIBODIES

Worse yet, the routine methods for detecting HIV antibodies are notoriously unreliable. Commercial HIV antibody tests are neither standardized nor reproducible. The test results mean different things in different laboratories and in different countries.

For example, a person who tests positive in Africa can be negative when tested in Australia, and a person who tests negative in Canada can become positive when tested in Africa. The same sample of blood tested in nineteen different laboratories got nineteen different results on the Western blot test (which tests for the presence of specific proteins).

"In short, the oft-stated claim that the HIV antibody test possesses high sensitivity and specificity is based on a comparison with the clinical manifestations of AIDS, or with CD4 cell count, which is poorly correlated with disease state," Rasnick remarks. "Importantly, the sensitivity and specificity of the HIV antibody test were not determined by a comparison with the presence of HIV itself—the usual reference standard."[3]

There are more than seventy documented ways that a person who has never been in contact with HIV can have false-positive antibodies to the virus.[4,5] These include naturally occurring antibodies, passive immunization, tuberculosis, lupus, kidney failure, hemodialysis, alpha interferon therapy, flu, flu vaccination, Herpes simplex I and II, pregnancy, rheumatoid arthritis, hepatitis, hepatitis B vaccination, tetanus vaccination, organ transplantation, anticollagen antibodies, autoimmune diseases, cancers, blood transfusions, multiple myeloma, hemophilia, Stevens-Johnson syndrome, and heat-treated specimens. (See also the chapter "Vaccinating People Against Their Own Genes.")

Newer antibody tests give more reproducible results. But the important question, says Rasnick, is whether the results of any HIV antibody test are a reliable indication of infection with HIV, and whether a positive result means that a person will eventually develop AIDS and die (see the chapter "Surviving and Thriving with HIV").

HIV ANTIBODIES DO NOT CORRELATE WITH AIDS DISEASE

HIV antibodies are just one of the "surrogate markers" for AIDS. There are two others: the CD4 cell count, which is the number of T-lymphocytes (a kind of immune cell) in the blood that have the CD4 marker (a particular protein on the cell surface), and the "viral load," or the level of virus detected with the polymerase chain reaction (PCR).[6]

From the beginning, doubt has arisen over whether CD4 T-lymphocytes could be a surrogate marker for AIDS disease.

The use of the CD4 T-cell counts as a surrogate marker of disease progression was also criticized by the authors of the Concorde study, the largest clinical trial evaluating the use of the anti-HIV drug zidovudine, known as AZT. They concluded, "The small but highly significant and persistent difference in CD4 count between the groups was not translated into a significant clinical benefit."[7]

Thomas Fleming and co-workers have stated the case even more baldly: "Predictions having an accuracy of approximately 50 percent, such as the accuracy seen with the CD4 count in the HIV setting, are as uninformative as a toss of a coin." With regard to clinical trials and FDA approval of anti-HIV drugs, Fleming and DeMets have warned that surrogate endpoints, such as CD4 cell count and viral load, are "rarely, if ever, adequate substitutes for the definitive clinical outcome in phase III trials."[8] Phased clinical trials are research studies that test new drugs or treatments to see how well they work on people. In the United States they are overseen by the Food and Drug Administration, and are conducted in a series of steps, called phases, each phase designed to answer a separate research question. Phase I tests the drug or treatment in a small group of people for the first time to evaluate its safety, determine a safe dosage range, and identify side effects. Phase II tests the drug or treatment on a larger group of people to see if it is effective and to further evaluate its safety. Phase III tests the drug or treatment on large groups of people to confirm its effectiveness, monitor side effects, compare it to commonly used treatments, and collect information that will allow the drug or treatment to be used safely.

A summary result from a 1993 state-of-the-art conference had previously concluded that the effect of treatment based on monitoring the most popular surrogate, CD4 cell count, did not accurately predict the effect of treatment on the clinical outcomes, that is, progression to AIDS or time to death.[9] Nevertheless, with the exception of the early AZT clinical trials, all subsequent anti-HIV drug trials and FDA approvals have relied exclusively on the measurements of these surrogate markers and not on the real clinical outcomes, such as morbidity and mortality, which are what matter most to most people.

A year later, Fleming stated:

> It is very apparent one cannot simply consider establishment of statistically significant treatment effects on CD4 cell counts to be a valid surrogate for either of the two clinical endpoints. When the progression to AIDS/death endpoint was positive, the CD4 endpoint appropriately was significantly positive in 7 of 8 trials; unfortunately however, the CD4 endpoint was significantly positive in 6 of 8 trials in which the progression to AIDS/death endpoint was negative. The relationship of CD4 effects and survival is even more unsatisfactory. The CD4 endpoint was significantly positive in only 2 of 4 trials in which the survival endpoint was positive; yet it was significantly positive in 6 of 7 trials in which the survival endpoint was negative. In three other trials, survival trends were observed which were in the opposite direction of significant treatment effects on CD4.[10]

HIV ANTIBODIES POORLY CORRELATED WITH HIV LOAD

The well-recognized problems with the CD4 count eventually led to its being replaced by the PCR viral-load test as the primary surrogate marker to be used in anti–HIV-drug clinical trials. But the viral-load test has its own problems—so much so that the company selling the test, Roche, has indicated on its label that its "AMPLICOR HIV-1 MONITOR Test is not intended to be used as a screening test for HIV or as a diagnostic test to confirm the presence of HIV infection."

Many "false positives" or "false negatives" have been found with the PCR test, depending on whether it is correlated with the presence of HIV antibodies. It has been widely criticized as lacking in sensitivity, specificity, and reproducibility.

One individual, for example, tested positive with PCR but was negative for HIV antibodies. So the patient's viral load of 100,000 (copies of the virus fragment per milliliter of blood) was renamed "false-positive" before extensive PCR testing in several laboratories returned the "right" answer: negative.[11] Another research group had noted several years earlier: "False-positive and false-negative results were observed in all laboratories";[12] concordance with HIV antibodies ranged between 40 and 100 percent.

The techniques for detecting cell-free HIV DNA (HIV DNA not contained within cells) simply "lacked adequate sensitivity, specificity and reproducibility for widespread clinical applications," wrote a third research team. "In any event, the levels of viral (and cellular) DNA in serum appear to be so low that reproducible detection, even with the use of PCR, is not currently possible."[13] That remains true to this day.

Rasnick sums up: "Simply put: the AIDS surrogate markers are being abused. These surrogate markers are causing a great deal of harm by labelling people with myriad diseases and conditions—even healthy people who only have antibodies to HIV—as having incurable AIDS, which is said to be invariably fatal. The surrogate markers are also being used to obtain FDA approval of clinically ineffective AIDS chemotherapies that are highly toxic and even lethal if taken long enough."[14]

AIDS and HIV

DOES HIV CAUSE AIDS? IS AIDS A SINGLE DISEASE?
DO ANTIVIRAL DRUGS REALLY HELP?

AIDS AS COMMONLY DEFINED

According to the *Medline Plus Medical Encyclopedia*, AIDS (acquired immune deficiency syndrome) is the final and most serious stage of human immunodeficiency virus (HIV) disease. HIV causes AIDS. The virus attacks the immune system and leaves the body vulnerable to a variety of life-threatening illnesses and cancers.[1]

HIV is transmitted through sexual contact, through blood (via blood transfusions) or needle sharing (among recreational intravenous drug-users), and from mother to child in pregnancy or during nursing.

The Centers for Disease Control has defined AIDS as beginning when a person with HIV infection has a CD4 cell count below 200. It is also defined by numerous opportunistic infections and cancers that occur in the presence of HIV infection.

The symptoms of AIDS are primarily the result of opportunistic infections.

Common symptoms are fevers, sweats (particularly at night), swollen glands, chills, weakness, and weight loss.

The AIDS-related infections and cancers that people with AIDS acquire as their CD4 count decreases include:

- **CD4 count below 350/μl:** herpes simplex virus, causing ulcers in the mouth or genitals; tuberculosis; oral or vaginal thrush due to

11

yeast infection; herpes zoster, causing ulcers over a discrete patch of skin; non-Hodgkin's lymphoma or cancer of the lymph glands.

- **CD4 count below 200/μl:** *Pneumocystis carinii* pneumonia; *Candida esophagitis* (painful yeast infection of the esophagus).
- **CD4 count below 100/μl:** Cryptococcal meningitis (infection of the brain by this fungus); AIDS dementia; *Toxoplasmosis* encephalitis (infection of the brain by this parasite frequently found in cat feces); progressive multifocal leukoencephalopathy (a viral disease of the brain caused by the JC virus, a polyoma virus named after the initials of the patient from whom it was originally isolated, that results in a quick decline in cognitive and motor functions); wasting syndrome (extreme weight loss and anorexia).
- **CD4 count below 50/μl:** *Mycobacterium avium* infection (a blood infection by a bacterium related to tuberculosis); cytomegalovirus infection (a viral infection that can affect almost any organ system, especially the eyes).

There is currently no cure for AIDS. However, several treatments are available that can delay the progression of disease for many years and improve the quality of life of those who have developed symptoms. Antiviral therapy suppresses the replication of HIV in the body. A combination of several antiretroviral agents, termed highly active antiretroviral therapy (HAART), has been highly effective in reducing the number of HIV particles in the bloodstream (as measured by a blood test called the viral load). This can help the immune system bounce back for a while and improve T-cell counts.

However, HIV tends to become resistant in patients who do not take their medications every day. Also, certain strains of HIV mutate easily and may become resistant to HAART especially quickly.

Treatment with HAART is not without complications. HAART is a collection of different medications, each with its own side-effect profile. Some common side effects are nausea, headache, weakness, malaise, and fat accumulation on the back and abdomen ("buffalo hump," or lipodystrophy). When used over the long term, these medications may increase the risk of heart attack by affecting fat metabolism.

Medications are also used to prevent opportunistic infections (such as *Pneumocystis carinii* pneumonia) and can keep AIDS patients healthier for long periods.

"HIV IS NOT THE CAUSE OF AIDS"

Dr. Peter Duesberg is a professor of molecular biology at the University of California at Berkeley, a member of the National Academy of Sciences, and a recipient of the 1985 Outstanding Investigative Grant from the National Institutes of Health. He was tipped as a Nobel candidate for his work on viral oncogenes (genes causing cancer).

But all that came to a crashing end in 1987, when he published a paper claiming that HIV did not cause AIDS, contrary to what the scientific community had come to believe (see above), but was instead the result of drug use.[2] He soon lost all his research grants, but that has not silenced him.

Ironically, Duesberg's hypothesis was generally held before the idea that HIV caused AIDS became accepted (see box).

Within a few years of Duesberg's paper, HIV-negative AIDS cases began to turn up, and people started to take notice of his theory, which he has refined over the years together with his colleague David Rasnick and others.

In a hefty review published in June 2003, Duesberg and Rasnick, together with Claus Koehnlein from Kiel, Germany, presented a long list of questions ("paradoxes") that the HIV-AIDS hypothesis cannot answer, or at least not satisfactorily according to the usual understanding of a viral disease.[3]

A Brief History of the HIV-AIDS Hypothesis

In 1981, a new epidemic began to strike male homosexuals and intravenous drug users in the United States and Europe. The U.S. Centers for Disease Control (CDC) termed the epidemic *AIDS*, for acquired immunodeficiency syndrome.

Between 1981 and 1984, leading researchers, including those from the CDC, suggested that recreational drug use was the cause of AIDS. But in 1984, U.S. government researchers proposed that a virus, now termed human immunodeficiency virus (HIV), was the cause of the epidemic in the United States and Europe, and also in Africa. This hypothesis—that HIV causes AIDS—gained instant acceptance within the scientific community.

One major difficulty that AIDS dissidents have with the HIV-AIDS hypothesis is that HIV, unlike ordinary viruses responsible for disease, cannot readily be isolated from AIDS patients. The viral load measured in patients refers, not to actual virus present, but to the amount of viral fragments that can be detected after amplification by PCR.

But defenders of the HIV-AIDS hypothesis have no trouble at all acknowledging that HIV is a strange new virus that can remain latent for years, being held in check by the body's immune system, which nevertheless finally succumbs to the virus.

The most contentious of Duesberg's claims is that AIDS is not contagious and is not sexually transmitted. That, his infuriated critics say, simply encourages people to have unprotected sex and to use dirty needles for injecting drugs, both of which would expose them to high risks of infection with HIV and a host of other disease agents besides. Yet that is perhaps the single point on which Duesberg and Rasnick are most adamant. Rasnick has stated categorically to the author in an e-mail message, "I want to stress that AIDS is not contagious, sexually transmitted or caused by HIV or any other virus." And he is able to cite at least as many papers to support his thesis as his opponents can to refute him.

"HIV does not cause AIDS, it is just a harmless passenger virus," insist Duesberg and his colleagues. (A passenger virus is a virus that happens to be present in some people but is not responsible for disease.) The WHO (World Health Organization) estimates that 34.3 million people were HIV-positive worldwide in 2000, yet only 1.4 percent developed AIDS. Similarly, in 1985, only 1.2 percent of the 1 million U.S. citizens with HIV developed AIDS.

Defenders of the HIV-AIDS hypothesis will readily admit that the progression from HIV infection to AIDS disease may indeed take years, but they say it will almost invariably happen.

Like all passenger viruses, Duesberg and Rasnick explain, HIV is inherited—that is, transmitted from mother to offspring—but is not infectious. AIDS disease in infants and children, according to Duesberg and Rasnick, results from prenatal consumption of recreational and anti-HIV drugs by unborn babies through their mothers. That too is a very contentious claim.

Duesberg and colleagues charge that "the HIV-AIDS hypothesis has remained entirely unproductive" to this day. There is as yet no anti–HIV/AIDS vaccine, no effective prevention, and not a single AIDS patient who has ever been cured. Those, they say, are "the hallmarks of a flawed hypothesis."

A much more productive hypothesis, according to Duesberg and Rasnick, is that AIDS is a collection of chemical epidemics caused by recreational drugs and anti-HIV drugs, and by malnutrition.

THE DURBAN DECLARATION

Duesberg is by no means a lone voice. The growing number of AIDS dissidents within the scientific community posed such a threat to the establishment that a remarkable declaration was made in Durban, South Africa, as thousands were gathering for the Thirteenth International AIDS Conference in July 2000. The declaration began: "HIV causes AIDS. Curbing the spread of this virus must remain the first step towards eliminating this devastating disease."[4]

The declaration, published in *Nature*, was signed by over five thousand people, including Nobel prizewinners; directors of leading research institutions, scientific academies, and medical societies, such as the U.S. National Academy of Sciences; the Max Planck Institutes; the Pasteur Institute in Paris; the Royal Society of London; the AIDS Society of India; and the National Institute of Virology in South Africa.

At the time, President Thabo Mbeki of South Africa had assembled a panel, known as the Presidential AIDS Advisory Panel, which included Duesberg and Rasnick, among other AIDS dissidents, together with many scientists holding the conventional view. Duesberg and Rasnick were among the eleven co-authors who signed a rebuttal to the Durban Declaration, published in *Nature* correspondence, stating that they "reject as outrageous" the attempt to outlaw open discussion of alternative viewpoints; it was an act of intolerance "which has no place in any branch of science."[5]

The full report of the Presidential AIDS Advisory Panel published a year later makes fascinating reading.[6] It is the best available summary of the complex debate over all aspects of AIDS, from causation to therapy. Unfortunately, none of the scientific papers cited by the panel members during the debate was included in the report.

AIDS IS A COLLECTION OF DISPARATE DISEASES

The starting point to this controversy is the disparate nature of the diseases that have been lumped together as AIDS. Even a staunch defender of the HIV-AIDS hypothesis, Helene Gayle, then director of the Centers for Disease Control's National Center of HIV, STD, and TB Prevention, and now director of the Bill and Melinda Gates Foundation's HIV, TB, and Reproductive Health Program, admitted at the end of the Presidential AIDS Advisory Panel debate that there is a general lack of standardization of the definition of AIDS throughout the world.[6] After fifteen years of research, there is no "gold standard" against which to measure the accuracy and reliability of the data generated from the commonly used methods to diagnose HIV infection. The major task ahead, said Gayle, was to develop such a gold standard.

Duesberg and colleagues show that different risk groups for AIDS disease have different conglomerates of AIDS-defining conditions. While Duesberg believes the AIDS disease does exist, Rasnick has argued consistently that AIDS does not exist and that it would "disappear instantaneously if all HIV testing was outlawed and the use of antiviral drugs terminated."

For example, Kaposi's sarcoma and *Pneumocystis* pneumonia are highly representative diseases among male homosexuals diagnosed with AIDS. But both conditions are absent or rare among African AIDS cases. Similarly, tuberculosis is highly represented among Africans but rare among European male homosexuals. More tellingly, hemophiliacs, who risk infection from blood transfusions, have no highly representative diseases at all, only two common infections—yeast and *Pneumocystis* pneumonia—thereby distinguishing them from all other risk groups.

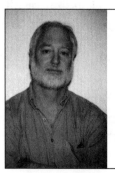

David Rasnick: "AIDS will disappear instantaneously if all HIV testing was outlawed and the use of antiviral drugs terminated."

AIDS AND RECREATIONAL DRUGS

At least thirty-five published studies up to 2002 have linked illicit recreational use of drugs such as nitrite and other inhalants, amphetamines, cocaine, heroin, and steroids with AIDS.

Shortly after the AIDS epidemics in the United States and Europe began, researchers found that illicit psychoactive and aphrodisiac drugs consumed in massive doses were the common factors and probable causes of AIDS. Drugs such as those listed above, plus lysergic acid (LSD), had become widely available and popular in the United States and Europe in the drug explosion during and after the Vietnam war, which coincided with the era of "gay liberation."

Recreational drug use rose steeply from 1980 to a peak between 1990 and 1995 and thereafter declined due to government crackdowns. The time course of the drug explosion correlates well with the number of AIDS cases, which rose from zero in 1980 to a sharp peak between 1992 and 1993 before declining sharply. Data from the CDC for 1983 showed that all 120 male homosexuals identified at that time as at risk for AIDS and 50 with AIDS were drug users. Consequently, many AIDS researchers favored the hypothesis that drug use or "lifestyle" was the cause of AIDS well into the 1990s.[7]

AFRICAN "EPIDEMIC" CAUSED BY POVERTY

In contrast, the African epidemic is caused by poverty—malnutrition and lack of drinkable water[8,9]—which is consistent with its random distribution in the population. According to some researchers, it is the same traditional diseases of the poor reclassified as AIDS (see the chapter "The African AIDS Epidemic").

The problems begin with the diagnosis of AIDS, which, in Europe and the United States, although not in Africa, is based on methods of detecting anti-HIV antibodies that are poorly standardized and prone to false positives, and also poorly correlated with the presence of the virus or other surrogate markers of AIDS disease, such as the level of CD4 cells (see "What Is AIDS Disease?"). According to Duesberg, African studies of patients diagnosed clinically as having AIDS showed that 50 percent were later found to be HIV-negative, that is, free of anti-HIV antibodies.[10]

African AIDS cases also have a different conglomerate of "AIDS-defining" diseases compared to other risk groups (see above).

AIDS CAUSED BY ANTI-AIDS DRUGS

Most if not all HIV-positive individuals with no sign of AIDS disease would remain healthy, according to Duesberg, especially if they avoid anti-HIV drugs like AZT and newer cocktails.

Since 1987, thousands of U.S. citizens and Europeans with AIDS, and since 1990, even larger numbers of healthy HIV-positive people, have been placed on lifetime prescriptions of toxic drugs like azidothymidine (AZT), which terminates DNA synthesis, and protease inhibitors aimed at suppressing assembly of the virus. Since 1996, DNA chain-terminators were mixed with HIV protease inhibitors in drug cocktails.

By 2002, more than 450,000 U.S. citizens were taking drug cocktails to prevent or cure AIDS, and well over half of them were clinically healthy at the time they started the anti-HIV drugs. The healthy HIV-positives were treated according to the slogan, "Time to hit HIV, early and hard," introduced by AIDS researcher David Ho in an article published in the *New England Journal of Medicine* in 1995.[11]

Duesberg and colleagues cited at least sixty-three scientific papers documenting diseases and death in HIV-positive people who had been placed on anti-HIV drugs over and above those in untreated controls. The conditions include AIDS-defining ones like immunodeficiency, leukopenia (low white blood cell count), fever, dementia, weight loss, lymphoma, and diarrhea; plus a host of other conditions that are non-AIDS-defining: anemia, neutropenia (low neutrophil count), nausea, lipodystrophy (redistribution of body fat), muscle atrophy, mitochondrial dysfunction (abnormal energy metabolism), hepatitis, birth defects, nephritis (inflammation of the kidney), lactic acidosis (excess lactic acid in the blood), and heart infarct (heart tissue damage due to obstruction of blood flow).

Similarly, at least twelve papers describe diseases and death in HIV-negative human babies and in HIV-negative animals treated with anti-HIV drugs before and after birth. The HIV-negative babies were born to mothers who had all been treated with AZT, which was found to reduce the natural transmission of HIV by 50 percent to 70 percent.

When HIV-infected infants born to mothers taking AZT during pregnancy were examined, the results showed that the children were 1.8 times more likely to develop severe disease, 2.4 times more likely to have severe immune suppression, and 3.2 times more likely to die than those HIV-infected infants born to mothers who did not take AZT.[12]

There is little doubt that the drugs are associated with numerous side effects, including those that are AIDS-defining. Evidence of toxicities accumulated throughout the late 1990s and finally led the U.S. government to appoint a panel of AIDS researchers to review the situation. In 2001, it issued recommendations to restrict prescriptions of anti-HIV drugs, suggesting that "treatment for the AIDS virus be delayed as long as possible for people without symptoms because of increased concerns over toxic effects of the therapy."[13]

The toxicities of anti-HIV drugs will be dealt with in more detail in the chapter "Anti-HIV Drugs Do More Harm Than Good."

WHY NOT TEST DUESBERG'S CHEMICAL HYPOTHESIS?

Although there is extensive circumstantial evidence to support Duesberg's chemical hypothesis, at least for some significant population of patients diagnosed with AIDS, it is difficult to prove without appropriate long-term controlled trials of antiviral drugs.

If Duesberg and his colleagues are right, they claim, "AIDS would be entirely preventable by banning anti-HIV drugs, by publicizing that recreational drugs cause AIDS and by adequate nutrition (see "Selenium Conquers AIDS"). Moreover, many AIDS patients could still be saved from fatal damage by drug intoxication, if their AIDS-defining diseases were treated with time-proven, disease-specific medications."

If they are wrong, many AIDS sufferers who could benefit from anti-HIV therapy will be misled, although this problem can be addressed by much more closely monitored and selective use of anti-HIV drugs.

Many researchers who think that HIV does cause AIDS admit that progression to disease—defined by low CD4 cell count and high viral load—can vary, and can be significantly affected by co-factors including recreational intravenous drug use and malnutrition. Others believe that HIV is necessary, although not sufficient, for causing AIDS disease. Dr. Veljko Veljković, an AIDS virologist in Belgrade, Yugoslavia, says,

"AIDS is a syndrome, and its different manifestations in different risk groups are not surprising because co-factors, which play an important role in AIDS development, are different." Thus, toxic chemicals and drugs may be among the co-factors that trigger the AIDS disease. Many co-factors induce the production of cytokines (proteins acting as chemical messengers produced by immune cells) and can suppress the immune system independent of HIV.

So why do current AIDS researchers not investigate or even consider the role of chemicals in AIDS, or study other non-HIV-AIDS theories to solve the AIDS dilemma?

Duesberg and colleagues blame "the structure of the large, government-sponsored research programs that dominate academic research since World War II," which favors an establishment that can impose sanctions on dissenters via the peer-review system.[14] The most powerful of the sanctions imposed are denial of funding and of publication.

Peer review is left to anonymous experts who do not fund applications that challenge their own interests. The review paper by Duesberg, Koehnlein, and Rasnick was blocked twice in the course of more than three years by the peer-review process in two separate journals before it finally appeared in print.

Perhaps the biggest hurdle to resolving the controversy is the failure of both sides to acknowledge the full complexity of the immune response. The proposal that recreational and toxic anti-HIV drugs, as well as malnutrition, can all undermine the immune system to produce immune deficiency syndromes is quite persuasive. But it may not be wise to exclude something like HIV that could target the immune cells directly (see "HIV and Latent Viruses").

The African AIDS Epidemic

AN ESTIMATED 26.6 MILLION PEOPLE IN SUB-SAHARAN AFRICA ARE
LIVING WITH HIV/AIDS, ACCORDING TO OFFICIAL FIGURES.
BUT CRITICS SAY THESE STATISTICS ARE NOTHING MORE THAN
HYPE SHROUDED IN SMOKE AND MIRRORS.

A MATTER OF DEFINITION

Being HIV-positive is the usual requirement for an AIDS diagnosis, but testing for HIV is something of a misnomer in Africa, where no HIV test is required to make an AIDS diagnosis. That is because in October 1985 a conference of public health officials, including representatives of the CDC and WHO, met in Bangui, Central Africa, to agree on a diagnostic definition of AIDS in Africa.

This definition was designed to allow clinicians to identify AIDS patients and to begin counting them seriously. The Bangui definition is: "prolonged fevers for a month or more, weight loss of over 10 percent and prolonged diarrhoea."[1] Agreeing to this definition has meant that traditional African diseases linked to poverty, war, famine, tropical climate, open latrines, and contaminated water are all neatly relabeled AIDS diseases. The consensus on Bangui is that "it has proved useful in areas where no testing is available." But as Charles Gilks pointed out in the *British Medical Journal* as early as 1991, "Persistent diarrhoea with weight loss can be associated with ordinary enteric parasites and bacteria." And, "In countries where the incidence of TB is high, substantial numbers of people reported as having AIDS may not in fact have AIDS."[2]

Since 1993, endemic diseases such as tuberculosis have been included as AIDS-defining illnesses, and in 2002, WHO dropped TB down its world's-greatest-killer list and moved AIDS up as the leading cause of death. The Statistical Assessment Service at George Mason University suggested that this was an attempt to "shift huge chunks of death around."[3] Cervical cancer has recently been added to the list of AIDS-defining diseases, which is easy to treat if detected quickly, but life threatening if not.

A MATTER OF EXTRAPOLATION

Professor Charles Gershetker, a frequent visitor to Africa as part of his research for California State University, discovered that some prenatal clinics were providing tests for HIV and collecting data. The problem with this is that pregnancy is one of the many conditions that can give a false-positive result with the standard enzyme-linked immuno-absorbent assay (ELISA) test for detecting anti-HIV antibodies. Other triggers for an incorrect result are recent vaccination and diseases such as hepatitis, influenza, malaria, and TB.

So the yearly "HIV-positive" results returned from 4,000 pregnant women were extrapolated by WHO's epidemiological computer to represent the entire population's burden of AIDS, male and female, young and old.

AIDS dissident Professor Jens Jerndal from the Group for the Scientific Reappraisal of the HIV-AIDS Hypothesis suggests that statistics are illusionist tricks to inflate the numbers of AIDS sufferers to inspire sufficient terror or panic in the general population to enable the introduction of mandatory medical interventions, or constraints on freedom of movement or behavior by those in power.[4] And for that, presenting the cumulative figure of those suffering from AIDS has more impact than reporting the number of new cases in a year, which would give a more accurate picture of the epidemic.

A MATTER OF MISDIAGNOSIS

The practice of widening the definitions of diseases diagnosed as AIDS also concerns Jerndal. At least twenty-nine different illnesses that existed before AIDS are considered as AIDS when they are accompanied by an

HIV-positive test. But there are more than sixty different conditions that can cause a positive result that bear no relation to HIV or AIDS (see "What Is AIDS Disease?"). Jerndal's message is that the world has been sold the unproven HIV-causes-AIDS dogma along with a fatal drug regime of conventional medicine that goes with it.

Misdiagnosis can have a devastating effect on the life of a patient, and aside from inaccurate results, a positive test for HIV is by no means predictive of the development of AIDS.[5] But so far no real distinction is made between testing HIV-positive and being diagnosed with AIDS.[6] Worse still, in Africa, an AIDS diagnosis can mean existing treatment is withheld altogether because of the entirely unjustified fatal prognosis attached to the illness.

A MATTER OF INFLATED STATISTICS

In whose interests would be the creation of numbers of people suffering from a fatal disease in epic proportions? In the United States in 2000, under President Clinton, AIDS in Africa, not in the United States, was declared a matter of national security. It was suggested that while AIDS was confined to the homosexual community in the United States, it was containable; but once heterosexual transmission had been established in Africa, everyone had a reason to panic, and AIDS budgets soared.[7]

Africans are being unfairly labeled as sexually promiscuous, reckless people while the key issue of poverty remains ignored. Statistics report HIV rates of infection as high as 25 percent in some African countries, and more women than men are infected.[8] World Bank statistics for those living with AIDS in sub-Saharan Africa are at 29.4 million, while in Cairo, Egypt, a short boat trip down the river, there are 215 cases of HIV/AIDS in a population of 65 million.[9]

U.N. antipoverty strategies that promised to halve debts in sub-Saharan Africa by 2015 are now, according to U.K. Chancellor Gordon Brown, more likely to reach their goal in 2047. Under the auspices of the World Bank and the International Monetary Fund, $2.5 billion is transferred from sub-Saharan African banks into foreign banks and creditors' accounts every year. A further blow is President Bush's proposal to cut core funding to Africa. Gordon Brown and singer Bono are calling for a doubling in cash aid to Africa.[10]

A MATTER OF POVERTY

People are dying of diseases in Africa caused by inadequate living conditions, and they deserve help now to improve quality of life, primarily through access to clean water and good nutrition. Constructive help, such as sustainable agricultural plans, would enable Africans to feed themselves.[11] Assistance like this could replace the manipulative measures of foisting U.S. tax-credit goods on African states. While thousands starved, pharmaceutical companies made "donations" of appetite stimulants to Sudan and silicone implants to Malawi. These companies then claimed tax credits for their useless gifts, and the recipient countries had to pay to dispose of them.[12]

It is unlikely that attaching emerging and traditional diseases to an AIDS definition is useful for tackling the key problems of malnutrition and sanitation, but it would encourage the use of pharmaceutical drugs. Costs for conventional drugs are still prohibitive for many Africans, and purchasing governments incur even greater debts to the World Bank. For any drug therapy to be truly successful, it must be used in tandem with adequate nutrition and sanitary conditions.

MISAPPLIED THERAPY

One of the most recent combination therapy drugs is called nevirapine; it is a nonnucleoside reverse transcriptase inhibitor (NNRTI), which reduces the viral load in HIV infection. It is causing neuropsychiatric side effects in patients with HIV who have no history of mental illness.[13] Three patients undergoing treatment developed psychotic reactions to the drug. Two made impulsive suicide attempts after suffering command hallucinations (hallucinations of being commanded to act), while the third experienced persecutory delusions and depressive thoughts after starting nevirapine. Physical side effects include hepatotoxicity, gastrointestinal symptoms, and dermatological reactions.

FACING THE FACTS

Leading AIDS dissident Dr. David Rasnick, a designer of protease inhibitors, used in the treatment of HIV infection, is confident that protease inhibitors can help reduce viral load but is unconvinced that HIV causes AIDS. He said in an interview for the *San Francisco Herald* in October 2000:

> In fact, I'm pretty sure right now there's no such thing as an AIDS epidemic in Africa, from my previous two trips last May and this July. The reason I say that in brief is that we've looked and looked and asked people, the government ministers, we asked the director of the medical research council in South Africa, the Centers for Disease Control in the U.S., everybody we could ask, "What are the numbers of AIDS cases in South Africa and how many AIDS deaths?" No answer at all. Zero. To this date we do not have an answer to that, and in fact, I don't think there is any such thing as AIDS going on in South Africa. It's just the same old things that Africans have been suffering and dying from for generations due to poverty, malnutrition, poor sanitation, bad water, that sort of thing. We're calling it AIDS now, instead of by the old-fashioned names that were more honest.[14]

Professor P. Addy, head of clinical microbiology at the University of Science and Technology in Kumasi, Ghana, backs up the opinions of AIDS dissidents. He says: "I've known for a long time that AIDS is not a crisis in Africa as the world is being made to understand. . . . The West came out with those frightening statistics on AIDS in Africa because it is unaware of certain social and clinical conditions. In most of Africa infectious diseases, particularly parasitic infections, are common. And these are the conditions that can easily compromise or affect one's immune systems." He concludes, "The diagnosis itself, merely being told you have AIDS, is enough to kill, and is killing people."[15]

The Ugandan Success Story

UGANDA IS WIDELY REGARDED AS AN **HIV/AIDS** SUCCESS STORY, BUT IT HAS BEEN WIDELY MISINTERPRETED AND GROSSLY EXAGGERATED.

DIRE PREDICTIONS NOT BORNE OUT

Dire predictions about the AIDS epidemic in Africa and Uganda were made as far back as 1984 on the cover of *Newsweek* magazine: "Can Africa be saved?" Two years later, the magazine ran the story again, headed "Africa in the Plague Years"; the article observed, "Nowhere is the disease more rampant than in the Rakai region of south-west Uganda, where 30 percent of the people are estimated to be seropositive."[1]

WHO agreed. It estimated that by mid-1991, 1.5 million Ugandans, or about 9 percent of the general population and 20 percent of the sexually active population, would have HIV infection.[2]

That estimate turned out to be a gross exaggeration.[3] WHO's own record shows that the African epidemic increased from 1984 until the early 1990s, similar to the American and European epidemics, but has since leveled off to about 75,000 cases a year. By 2001, the entire African continent had a total of 1,093,522 AIDS cases since 1984. During the same period, the population of sub-Saharan Africa had grown at an annual rate of about 2.6 percent per year, from 378 million in 1980 to 652 million in 2000.

A "SUCCESS" DECLARED

In fact, the proportion of people with HIV has been declining in Uganda since 1992, as reported in a number of surveillance sites around the country. The international community enthusiastically praises Uganda for its success in tackling the epidemic and urges other nations, especially those in Africa, to learn from Uganda.

Uganda seems indeed unique in Africa in the extent to which HIV is decreasing. Furthermore, as the first African country to identify individuals with AIDS and to establish a national response program, it sets an ideal example for other nations of how to deal with the disease.

"SUCCESS" BASED ON MISINFORMATION

However, many claims of the success in Uganda are based on selective pieces of information, which, according to Dr. Justin Parkhurst of the London School of Hygiene and Tropical Medicine, "have been falsely presented as representative of the nation as a whole."[4]

Such data have been used, for example, to claim that overall rates of HIV in Uganda have been reduced from 30 percent to 10 percent, a claim that has been reproduced in the National Strategic Framework for HIV Activities in Uganda and in the mass media. Statements such as these are probably based on data from government antenatal clinic surveillance sites, generally recognized as biased because they exaggerate recorded declines in prevalence of the disease, the proportion of people infected with HIV.

A second misinterpretation of data appears in the claims that *incidence* rates of HIV—the number of new cases each year—in Uganda have fallen, which are often based on the government surveillance data providing only estimates of prevalence rates.

Successful HIV prevention cannot be claimed until there is a decrease in incidence, says Parkhurst. Prevalence can decline while incidence remains stable or even increases, for example, if death rates of the HIV-infected population were to increase above the incidence rate. Indeed, the first significant data on declining incidence rates in Uganda was not presented until 2000, at the Durban International AIDS Conference in South Africa.

Nevertheless, there is growing evidence to suggest that the incidence of HIV across Uganda is declining. A fall in prevalence rates among the youngest age groups, especially fifteen- to nineteen-year-olds, at surveillance sites is considered a proxy measure of incidence. Individuals in this group have only recently become sexually active, so a decrease in prevalence among them is unlikely to be due to death from AIDS.

Young women in this age group attending antenatal clinics in central urban and western regions of the country have shown particularly pronounced declines in prevalence rates.

THE UGANDAN GOVERNMENT DESERVES MUCH OF THE CREDIT, BUT NOT ALL

Another frequent mistake is to attribute the decline in prevalence rates to a few interventions introduced by the Ugandan government.[5] The government is but one player in the fight against HIV. Hundreds of nongovernmental organizations (NGOs), religious groups, and community activists are also working to prevent the spread of HIV/AIDS in Uganda. The Ugandan government itself has widely acknowledged the roles that other groups have played in the fight against HIV, referring to them as partners in HIV prevention. Moreover, individuals may be changing their behavior independently of the intervention programs due to a growing general awareness of the effect of AIDS on friends or relatives, for example.

Intriguingly, many mathematical models predict that although prevalence rates will reflect declines in incidence, they will do so only after a time lag of seven years or more.[6] Hence, a decline in prevalence beginning in 1992 would correspond with a fall in incidence from the beginning of 1985, when Uganda was in the midst of its civil war and did not have any national HIV prevention program. David Rasnick of the University of California at Berkeley, one of the most outspoken and tireless AIDS dissidents, has commented on the same leveling off and decline in incidence in Europe and North America.[7] Could it simply be the natural progression of the disease epidemic?

"Nevertheless, other African nations have not seen similar declines in prevalence," Parkhurst said, "suggesting that Uganda alone must have acted in a way that changed the course of its HIV/AIDS epidemic."[8] He pointed out that the government has, for example, not only provided services such as education and blood screening across the country, but also "implemented a uniquely creative and strategic policy approach to enable non-state actors in their individually targeted messages of prevention."

The openness of Uganda is often mentioned; the Ugandan government included religious groups and NGOs in policy-recommending bodies such as the Uganda AIDS Commission, which has resulted in cooperative links and enabled wider participation between the governmental and nongovernmental groups. Nor did the government push controversial policies too strongly; for example, it quietly promoted condoms through social marketing channels, again including religious leaders in discussions.

Finally, the widely cited political leadership of the Museveni administration must be given due credit as a national government committed to addressing HIV/AIDS through all available channels.

UGANDAN SUCCESS REAL THOUGH EXAGGERATED

Uganda has indeed been successful in slowing the spread of HIV. But widely cited claims, such as the reduction of prevalence rates from 30 to 10 percent in four or six years, are unfounded. Today, the adult HIV prevalence rate is most likely much lower than 10 percent and continues to decline, but still there remains no evidence that the nation ever saw a 20 percent fall in prevalence rates. Such exaggerations may have resulted from pressure to present success stories to donors.[9]

In fact, the UNAIDS estimate for Uganda released at the Fifteenth International AIDS Conference in July 2004 is that 4.1 percent adults between fifteen and forty-nine years of age are living with HIV.[10]

AIDS Aid: Big Profit
for Pharma Giants

THE STRUGGLE FOR ACCESS TO CHEAP GENERIC ANTI-HIV DRUGS IN THIRD WORLD COUNTRIES CONTINUES.

GLOBAL INITIATIVES TO COMBAT AIDS
WITH ANTI-HIV DRUGS

President George Bush pledged $15 billion in 2003 to fight AIDS over the next five years. Philanthropic foundations, such as those of Bill and Melinda Gates and Bill Clinton, have also contributed their support. WHO launched its "three-by-five" initiative to supply anti-HIV drugs to 3 million people by 2005.

In 2003, the British government donated $452 million to combat AIDS, second after the United States, which gave $577 million. U.K. Secretary of State for International Development Hilary Benn announced a further £113 million (approximately $215 million) donation to UNAIDS and the U.N. Population Fund in July 2004. Other donors, including Germany, Japan, Canada, the European Union, the Netherlands, Norway, Australia, Ireland, Italy, and France gave a total of $1.64 billion.

It is estimated that $20 billion is needed by 2007. A large portion of the budget will be spent on providing anti-HIV drugs, which have been produced by big pharmaceutical companies and sold at greatly inflated prices to AIDS sufferers in rich countries.[1]

CHEAP GENERICS DENIED BY BUSH ADMINISTRATION

Thanks to modern combination drugs, more and more people suffering from AIDS in Europe and North America are now surviving the disease, so it is often said. Shouldn't this benefit be extended to AIDS sufferers in Africa and other countries in the developing world?

Cheap generic versions of the anti-HIV drugs costing a small fraction of the brand-name versions and validated by WHO are already in use in poor countries. But the United States, under pressure from pharmaceutical companies, is trying to undermine that practice.[2] They want the money promised by the Bush administration to help fight AIDS in the third world to be spent on purchase of their patented products, rather than the cheap generics selling for less than the £165 per patient per year price set by the pharmaceutical giants as a special concession to the third world.

The U.S. Department of Health and Human Services convened a conference in Botswana at the end of March 2004 to question WHO's approval process for generic drugs, but no agreement was reached.

GENERICS MEET STANDARDS

A study published in the journal *Clinical Infectious Disease* in May 2004 showed that generic antiviral drugs distributed in four developing countries met U.S. Pharmacopoeia (USP) standards. Researchers at the National Institutes of Health and the University of Alabama evaluated six different types of anti-HIV drugs obtained from doctors in Lithuania, South Africa, Jamaica, and Zambia.[3] All fell within the USP-approved efficacy range.

POOR COUNTRIES DEFIANT

Developing countries are defiant.[4] Thailand had begun selling its own locally produced antiretroviral drug in April 2003 at a cost of less than a dollar a day per patient. It combines in a single pill the strengths of the triple-drug cocktail of stavudine, lamivudine, and nevirapine, all of which are inhibitors of the reverse transcriptase enzyme necessary for viral replication.

India too has slashed the costs of AIDS drugs to $0.38 per patient a day for the triple-drug regimen, which is now being distributed in India. Thanks to Indian drug makers, the cost of the highly active antiretroviral therapy (HAART) plummeted in price last year. The treatment, which earlier cost thousands of dollars, can now be bought from Bombay-based Cipla and other generic companies for less than $250 a year.

In a further boost, research published in the *Lancet* suggests that a single dose of the three generic drugs is as effective as separate doses of the expensive brand-name drugs.

Ayanda Ntsaluba, director general of South Africa's foreign trade, said his government was looking to India for "practical solutions" to tackle AIDS.

About 440,000 people are on AIDS drugs in poor countries,[5] some 50,000 in Africa. The group of physicians Médecins Sans Frontières (MSF; Doctors Without Borders), which runs free AIDS treatment programs in Africa, currently gives them to some 9,000 patients.[6] In Zimbabwe, MSF treats patients for £109 ($207) to £136 ($259) a year, while a program run by the CDC uses brand-name drugs, after price reduction, at £325 ($618) per patient per year.

WTO VICTORY NOT IMPLEMENTED

After a protracted struggle, an agreement was finally reached in August 2003 at the World Trade Organization (WTO) conference at Cancun, Mexico, to allow developing countries to import generic drugs if the country confirms that it cannot manufacture them domestically.[7] But so far, only Mozambique, Malaysia, and Canada have adopted legislation to implement the agreement.

The Canadian Parliament adopted a bill in May 2004 that would amend its patent laws to permit the government to order the override of patents so as to allow certain pharmaceutical manufacturers to produce and export generic drugs for use in developing countries. But it seems that the battle is not yet over.

UNITED STATES TURNING AIDS INTO BIG BUSINESS

Under the WTO Agreement on Trade-Related Aspects of Intellectual Property Rights (TRIPS), the implementation of patent rules applying to drugs will start on January 2006; and countries that currently observe no patent rules will either cease to produce generic drugs or will price them above the purchasing power of the poor countries.

But on June 27, 2002, the WTO council responsible for intellectual property rights approved a decision extending the transition period—during which least-developed countries do not have to provide patent protection for pharmaceuticals—to 2016. It also approved a waiver that would exempt poor countries from having to provide exclusive marketing rights for any new drugs in the period when they do not provide patent protection. That waiver was to have been submitted to the WTO General Council for approval on July 8, 2002.

Uganda failed to take advantage of this waiver. Why? Uganda has apparently allowed its patent legal review process to be "mentored," and hence commandeered, by the U.S. Agency for International Development (USAID), according to advocates of drug access.[8]

Under the patent protection rules, if a country's health authority approves a new drug for sale, the patent applicant has to be given exclusive marketing rights for five years even though there is no patent. Nonetheless, the subsequent agreement negotiated in Cancun means that governments *can* issue compulsory licenses to allow other companies to make a generic copy of the patented product or use a patented process under license without the consent of the patent owner.

The United States, however, has been working to undermine the Cancun agreement. First, a huge proportion of the $15 billion the U.S. government has poured into the fight against AIDS will be spent to purchase U.S.-patented drugs, not the generic drugs promoted by WHO and the Global Fund for AIDS. Worse, the United States is now entering into bilateral agreements with developing countries that produce generic drugs to opt out of the August 2003 waiver agreement.

France's President Jacques Chirac attacked the Bush administration at the international AIDS conference in Bangkok in July 2004. Chirac accused the United States of blackmailing developing countries into giving up their right to produce cheap drugs for AIDS victims. He said there is a real problem of favorable trade deals being dangled before poor nations in return for those countries halting production of lifesaving generic drugs.

Not all African nations have allowed the United States to bully them into using patented drugs.[9]

Like Mozambique, many countries prefer generics because they can be combined in a fixed dose in one tablet, improving adherence to pill-taking schedules. So Mozambique, Namibia, and Rwanda, among others, are holding fast to generics.

Uganda, in contrast, finds its hands tied, and patients are already feeling the impact of using brand-name drugs distributed under President Bush's HIV/AIDS program. Warnings are regularly issued through the press that these FDA-approved antiretroviral treatments must be taken under close supervision of a medical practitioner. "And how is this to help our remote rural population who live miles away from the nearest dispensary?" asks Anne Mugisha Bwomezi, secretary of international and regional affairs, reform agenda, in an article entitled, "How US is turning AIDS into big business."[10]

In Maputo, Mozambique, health officials said that they were struck by the Americans' obsession with numeric goals. "To see an increase in numbers of people on antiretrovirals, that was their only concern," said Songane. "But this is a complex disease. We cannot judge the success of our fight just by the numbers of people on treatment."[11]

In April 2005, the Indian government passed a patent-amendment bill to make the country conform to the WTO TRIPS patent regime.[12] The amendment covers food, pharmaceutical, and agribusiness sectors and can be expanded over time to other sectors. India is the chief producer of cheap generic copies of patented drugs aimed at treating or preventing disease epidemics in the third world, such as AIDS, malaria, hepatitis and tuberculosis, which are sold at around 5 percent of the price charged by the big pharmaceutical corporations. This recent patent amendment has put an end to cheap generic drugs, with serious repercussions on the health of the poorest nations.

Anti-HIV Drugs Do More Harm Than Good

THE EFFICACY AND SAFETY OF CONVENTIONAL PHARMACEUTICAL DRUGS NEED CLOSER SCRUTINY AS HUGE GLOBAL INITIATIVES LAUNCHED TO TREAT AIDS IN AFRICA AND ELSEWHERE ARE LARGELY LINKED TO THE PURCHASE OF SUCH DRUGS.

DO ANTI-HIV DRUGS REDUCE AIDS DEATHS?

Although the pharmaceutical giants are concerned with profit rather than safety, it is worth noting that these drugs come with many acknowledged harmful side effects;[1] increasingly, people are asking whether the harm they do outweighs the benefits.

It is claimed that anti-HIV drugs extend life in AIDS sufferers, as the mortality rate from AIDS has been decreasing. This claim may be faulty, however, for at least two reasons, as David Rasnick suggests.[2] First, AIDS mortality was already going down before the combination drugs were introduced. Data from the CDC show that AIDS peaked in 1992 and has been decreasing steadily ever since.[3] The mortality rate from AIDS is dropping simply because AIDS has been declining in the United States since 1992, years before the introduction of the anti-HIV cocktail HAART. It has little to do with the effectiveness of HAART.

Second, the CDC redefined AIDS to include healthy people.[4] As of 1993, all a person needs to qualify as an AIDS case are results from two lab tests: antibodies to the virus, and fewer than 200 CD4 cells (cells expressing the surface marker CD4) per microliter of blood.

As a result, over half the people treated with anti-HIV drug cocktails in the United States since 1996 (the year the HIV protease-inhibitor cocktails became available) were healthy when they started taking the drugs. The mainstream AIDS press and AIDS researchers are crediting HAART with prolonging the lives of these healthy people. Sadly, these healthy people taking HAART don't stay healthy long. They eventually get sick and die if they stay on the drug cocktails long enough.

TOXICITIES OF ANTI-HIV DRUGS RAISE DOUBT OVER LIFETIME TREATMENT

A year after HAART was introduced, Dr. Jay Levy, a leading AIDS researcher from the University of California School of Medicine in San Francisco, had already expressed his concern over early treatment of people without symptoms,[5] which appears to have the effect of suppressing the immune system, leaving these people more vulnerable to the virus.

Researchers are now questioning whether AIDS patients should be kept on the drugs continuously for more than two years. In a study published in 2004, researchers in Necker Hospital in Paris concentrated on patients with HIV infection treated with HAART whose treatment was considered "highly successful." "Highly successful" was defined as attaining a reduced viral load within six months of starting the first HAART regimen and maintaining this lowered level for forty-eight months or more.

Of the 217 patients enrolled, 13 died, 19 were lost to follow-up, and only 41 (less than 20 percent) were considered "highly successful" and were followed up for more than forty-eight months. Of the 41, 2 died after sixty months, 1 of terminal liver failure and the other of lymphoma, but both still had undetectable plasma viral loads. All other patients were clinically well, except for the lipodystrophy syndrome, which was present in 58.5 percent.

The researchers concluded: "It is more and more difficult to imagine anti-HIV treatments as life-long prescriptions, given the side effects described in the long term, such as lipodystrophy (found here in nearly 60 percent of patients), metabolic disturbances, a possibly increased cardiovascular risk, mitochondrial toxicity and altered quality of life."

In other words, the inconvenience of very long-term treatment may outweigh the benefit of maintaining the CD4 cell count at a high level, and treatment beyond two to four years did not result in a significant further reduction of the viral load.[6]

It is now routine for patients to take "holidays" from the toxic drug treatments when their markers of AIDS disease warrant it. In January 2002, the Community Programs for Clinical Research on AIDS (CPCRA) in the United States announced the SMART Study (Strategies for Management of Antiretroviral Therapy), to be carried out by sixteen units in the CPCRA, plus five other sites in the United States and sites in Australia associated with the Australian National Centre in HIV Epidemiology and Clinical Research. The National Institute of Allergy and Infectious Diseases of the National Institutes of Health is sponsoring the study.[7]

The study will enroll 6,000 people above the age of thirteen over a three-year period. Participants will be followed for six to nine years to assess the risks and benefits of continuous treatment compared with "structured treatment interruptions," that is, using antiretroviral drugs episodically only when the participants' CD4 T-cell count drops below 250 cells/μl, and discontinued when the CD4 T-cell count rises above 350 cells/μl.

"This approach of not using antiretroviral medications when CD4+ T-cell counts are higher and when the risks of complications of HIV are low could have the advantage of reducing side effects, drug resistance and cost, while saving antiretroviral medication options for a time when the risk of complications from HIV begins to increase," said Dr. Wafaa El-Sadr, principal investigator at Harlem Hospital and Columbia University in New York and co-chair of the study.[8] Dr. James Neaton, principal investigator at the CPCRA Statistical Center at the University of Minnesota in Minneapolis and co-chair of the SMART study team, added, "The initiation of the SMART study marks an important turning point in HIV research."[9]

ANTI-HIV DRUGS

There are nineteen single drugs and two combination drugs approved by the Food and Drug Administration (FDA) for treating HIV/AIDS.[10] They fall into four classes.

The *DNA chain-terminators* include nucleoside analogs such as AZT, which were developed in the 1960s as cytotoxic (toxic to cells) chemotherapy for cancer. These drugs are not only inhibitors but also substrates of the human enzymes responsible for DNA synthesis. As substrates, the drugs are incorporated into growing DNA chains, thus terminating the chain, which kills or otherwise injures the cells. All the anti-HIV nucleoside analogs come with a "black-box" label (the FDA's most serious warning placed on the label of a prescription medicine) warning of severe life-threatening toxicities, which include profound general depression of the immune system, anemia, lactic acidosis, and liver damage, among numerous other unpleasant effects. The nonnucleoside analog nevirapine is no less toxic. It has its own black-box label warning of life-threatening liver toxicity and life-threatening skin reactions. These toxic chain-terminators are typically prescribed at high dosages—such as a 100 mg capsule five times a day—even to pregnant mothers.

The *HIV protease inhibitors* were designed to inhibit HIV assembly. Because no therapeutic effects were observed at low doses at which these inhibitors block HIV replication in the test tube, the "antiviral" doses prescribed are four to five orders of magnitude higher, that is, 1 to 2 g per day, which is at least fifty times what is needed to completely inhibit the essential enzyme intestinal aspartyl protease cathepsin D. Mice without cathepsin D develop anorexia, their thymus and spleen undergo massive destruction with severe loss of T- and B-cells, and they die about twenty-six days after birth. Other side effects include lipodystrophy (redistribution of body fat), elevated cholesterol and triglycerides, diarrhea, and metabolic disturbances.

HAART (highly active antiretroviral therapy) consists of drug cocktails containing AZT and other DNA chain-terminators supplemented with protease inhibitors. Severe side effects include liver failure, neutropenia, anemia, kidney failure, AIDS-defining conditions, and death.

Fusion inhibitors are a new class of drugs that act against HIV by preventing the virus from fusing with the cell in order to enter it. Only one has been approved so far, and it is approved for use only in people whose HIV has become resistant to available antiretrovirals. Side effects detected during clinical trials: itching, swelling, pain, tenderness, hardened skin and bumps at site of injection, serious allergic reaction in less than 1 percent of patients, and an increase in the rate of bacterial pneumonia.

DRUG RESISTANCE

The emergence of drug-resistant viruses has been keeping pace with the development of new antiviral drugs. HAART, the cocktail designed to overcome drug resistance, was introduced in 1996. A study published in July 2004 estimated that 76 percent of HIV-positive patients with virus in their blood—who received medical treatment in 1996 and survived to 1998—had resistance to one or more antiretroviral drugs.[11] The odds of resistance were significantly higher in patients with a history of antiretroviral drug use, advanced HIV disease, higher plasma viral load, and low CD4 cell counts.

A similar study published a year earlier tested 1,633 newly infected HIV-positive patients from seventeen European countries. At least 9.6 percent were resistant to at least one of the three types of antiretroviral drugs in use: 6.9 percent to nucleoside reverse-transcriptase inhibitors, 2.6 percent to nonnucleoside reverse-transcriptase inhibitors, and 2.2 percent to protease inhibitors.[12] Thus, people are more and more likely to become infected with drug-resistant viral strains, which would compromise drug treatment even before it begins.

Worse yet, there is no convincing evidence that these drugs actually work.

NO EVIDENCE THAT THE ANTI-HIV DRUGS WERE EFFECTIVE

The Durban Declaration of 2000 (see the chapter "AIDS and HIV") asserted that anti-HIV drugs "reduced the progression of AIDS mortality by 80 percent" and "delay the progression to AIDS," but these claims were not borne out by the evidence.[13]

The National Institutes of Health, in collaboration with the U.S. drug manufacturer Burroughs Wellcome, carried out a licensing study on AZT in 1987. The study showed that after four months on AZT, only one out of 145 AIDS patients died, whereas 19 out of 139 died in the control placebo group.[14,15]

However, among the survivors in the AZT group, 30 could be kept alive only with multiple blood transfusions because their red cells had been severely depleted. In addition, many AZT recipients had developed life-threatening bone-marrow suppression, neutropenia (low count of neutrophil white blood cells), macrocytosis (enlarged red blood cells associated with anemia), headaches, insomnia, and myalgia (muscle pain), which augured poorly for their future survival.

But based on this study, AZT was approved through a "fast track" process and licensed to Britain's largest multinational drug-supported charity, Wellcome Foundation,[16] thereby giving the multinational an effective monopoly over the treatment for AIDS and preventing other promising candidates from being developed for years.

The report on the largest placebo-controlled trial of immediate and deferred AZT treatment in symptom-free HIV-positive individuals, the U.K.-French Concorde study, was published in 1994. This study investigated 1,749 HIV-positive, mostly male homosexual subjects divided into untreated and AZT-treated subgroups for the onset of AIDS and death. It found AZT unable to prevent AIDS. On the contrary, AZT use was associated with an excess of life-threatening and other severe adverse events. It concluded, "The results of Concorde do not encourage the early use of zidovudine (AZT) in symptom-free HIV-infected adults."[17]

The new drug cocktails were no better. In a front-page article in *The New York Times* in 1997, Dr. Anthony Fauci, director of the National Institute of Allergy and Infectious Diseases (NIAID), was reported to have said, "There is an increasing percentage of people in whom, after a period of time, the virus breaks through. People do quite well for six months, eight months or a year, and after a while, in a significant proportion, the virus starts to come back."[18]

Fauci estimated that when these cases of "viral breakthrough" are accounted for, the failure rate of the new drug cocktails could be as high as 50 percent.

"Fauci's failure rate was really 100 percent in the AIDS cases that actually have symptoms of disease." Rasnick says.[19] That is because, since 1993, 50 percent of AIDS cases have no symptoms of the disease.[20]

The U.S. government finally set up an expert panel to review anti-HIV therapy in 2001. This led to recommendations to restrict the prescription of anti-HIV drugs and to delay treatment for the AIDS virus for as long as possible for people without symptoms, on account of the serious side effects.

The side effects mentioned include nerve damage, weakened bones, unusual accumulations of fat in the neck and abdomen (lipodystrophy), diabetes, and dangerously high levels of cholesterol and other lipids in the blood that could lead to heart disease.

NEW EVIDENCE OF RISKS FROM HAART

New evidence has emerged that HAART patients are at risk from both severe side effects as well as AIDS, with the risk from the former about twice that of the latter. A study published in December 2003 analyzed the data from five U.S. multicenter HAART trials that had a common system of reporting adverse events—AIDS events and deaths—between 1996 and 2001, and involved 2,947 patients followed up for a median of 20.7 months.[21]

A severe or life-threatening side effect was experienced by 675 individuals; 332 developed an AIDS-defining condition; and 272 died.

The cumulative percentage of patients with a severe or life-threatening side effect at month twelve was 15.6 percent, at month twenty-four 23.7 percent, and at month thirty-six 30.8 percent. The corresponding percentages for AIDS events were 7.3 percent, 10.8 percent, and 16.5 percent; while the percentages of deaths were 3.9 percent, 7.9 percent, and 13.1 percent.

The risk of severe or life-threatening side effects was significantly lower in younger patients (HR, or hazards ratio, 0.83 for every decade in years) and for patients who had never taken anti-HIV drugs before (HR 0.59), and increased for individuals with a history of intravenous drug use (HR 1.41), lower baseline CD4 cell count (HR 1.06 for every 100 cells per microliter), and a prior AIDS-defining illness (HR 1.22).

The most frequently reported side effects were associated with the liver. But women were at increased risk of severe or life-threatening neutropenia (HR 1.76), while African-Americans were at increased risk of neutropenia (HR 3.78), anemia (HR 2.46), and kidney-related events (HR 22.41). People of Latino origin had an increased risk of neutropenia (HR 2.75).

Of the 272 who died, 159 had both a severe life-threatening reaction and an AIDS-defining illness.

ANTI-HIV DRUGS REDUCE HIV TRANSMISSION IN PREGNANCY

Perhaps the most controversial issue is the use of anti-HIV drugs on the unborn. In 1994, the Pediatric AIDS Clinical Trial Group (PACTG) reported that giving AZT to a woman during pregnancy, labor, and the post-delivery period could decrease the mother-to-child transmission of HIV by 67.5 percent.[22] At eighteen months, 8.3 percent of infants born to mothers treated with AZT while pregnant became HIV-positive, compared with 25.5 percent of infants born to mothers not treated with AZT while pregnant.

The practice of giving AZT to mothers during pregnancy had already begun in the early 1990s; and since the PACTG study, AZT treatment was routinely recommended during the second half of pregnancy and during labor, and, for the newborn, for the first six weeks of life. This has led to a substantial decrease in the number of HIV-infected children in the developed countries.

Simplified regimens, adapted for use in Africa and South Asia, have also been reported to be effective in reducing the transmission of HIV to children by 50 percent. But there have been few follow-up studies on the children after birth.

FOLLOW-UP STUDIES REVEAL DAMAGE TO INFANTS

A research team from the coordinating Centres of the Italian Register for HIV Infection in Children compared infants who were HIV-infected from mothers receiving AZT (AZT+) during pregnancy with those from mothers receiving no AZT (AZT–) during pregnancy.[23]

The study included 216 infants infected with HIV; 38 were born to AZT+ mothers, and 178 were born to AZT– mothers. The two groups did not differ in the frequency of children receiving antiviral drugs at various times after birth. Because there was a rapid death rate in infants born to AZT+ mothers, analyses were limited to the first three years of life.

The results showed that the children born to AZT+ mothers were 1.8 times more likely to develop severe disease, 2.4 times more likely to have severe immune suppression, and 3.2 times more likely to die than those born to AZT– mothers.

Despite these findings against the use of AZT during pregnancy, which completely wiped out the supposed benefit of reducing HIV transmission, the researchers drew the conclusion that prenatal AZT treatment had failed and called for even more aggressive antiviral treatments applied earlier.

In another more recent study, 152 infants born to mothers taking no AZT during pregnancy were compared with 139 infants born to mothers who did take AZT. The rate of transmission of HIV was significantly reduced from 22.3 percent in infants from AZT– mothers to 12.2 percent in AZT+ mothers. But among the infected infants, rapid disease progression was 29.4 percent in the AZT– group compared with 70.6 percent in the AZT+ group.[24] In other words, 8.61 percent of the infants born to mothers given AZT during pregnancy progressed rapidly to AIDS disease, compared with 6.55 percent of the infants born to mothers not given AZT during pregnancy.

There has been only one large follow-up study of HIV-negative infants born to mothers treated with anti-HIV drugs during pregnancy, and it was carried out in France. A total of 1,754 children born to mothers exposed to AZT or other anti-HIV drugs as part of the mother's treatment during pregnancy were followed up. The researchers found eight children with mitochondrial dysfunction, all of whom were HIV-negative. Five, two of whom died, presented with delayed neurological symptoms, and three were symptom-free but had severe biological or neurological abnormalities. All children had abnormally low activities of one or more respiratory chain complexes (involved in energy metabolism in the mitochondrion).[25]

The researchers noted, "The symptoms in the children in our study were not specific, and may therefore have not been identified as toxic effects of treatment." They pointed to three children out of 107 in an earlier follow-up study with unexplained symptoms of the heart and the eye,[26] which could be related to mitochondrial dysfunction.

While the researchers did not call for an end to the prophylactic antiviral treatment of children in the uterus, they said pregnant women "should be informed of the potential effects associated with these treatments during pregnancy."

HIV-POSITIVE SURVIVORS WITHOUT DRUGS

Duesberg and colleagues[27] cited eleven published scientific papers documenting HIV-positive individuals surviving for more than ten years who had not used antiviral therapy. There are also many corroborating anecdotes, including reports on individuals who came off anti-HIV drugs because they had become very sick and went on to survive many years afterwards.

The mainstream AIDS research community has acknowledged the existence of long-term survivors of HIV infection as a "small minority" that show either no progression or slow progression to AIDS disease.

There are no official estimates on the proportion of HIV-infected people who will progress slowly to AIDS, or not progress at all. Among 539 men in San Francisco infected with HIV for at least ten years, 42 (8 percent) had CD4 counts above 500, who would be classified as nonprogressors. But 31 percent had not developed AIDS, which means that a substantial minority with low CD4 cell counts can remain well for long periods, something that researchers simply do not understand, nor do they know what proportion will stay well despite immune damage.[28] Another study found that of 579 gay men with CD4 counts below 200, 20 percent did not develop AIDS for three years.[29]

It has been debated whether there truly are any nonprogressors. But there is evidence that some people not only do not seem to progress to AIDS disease, they are able to control HIV infection with spontaneous decreases in HIV DNA levels.

Ongoing studies are comparing slow and fast progressors to identify the role of co-factors including lifestyle. A recent report suggests that slow progression to AIDS disease is associated with rare variants in human leukocyte antigens (HLAs) involved in the immune response against viruses and bacteria.

Claus Koehnlein initiated a study in 1985 of thirty-six AIDS patients in Kiel, Germany, who had volunteered to abstain from anti-HIV treatments.[30] Only three have died since their anti-HIV antibodies were first detected—two after sixteen years and one after ten years. *Most have recovered from their initial AIDS-indicator symptoms.*

By contrast, 63 percent of all German AIDS patients (11,700 of 18,700), most of which were treated since 1987 with anti-HIV drugs, had died during the same period.[31]

It now appears that abstaining from anti-HIV treatment is one major factor contributing to long-term survival in people infected with HIV, as we shall see in the next chapter.

Surviving and Thriving
with HIV

WHILE MANY WHO TEST HIV-POSITIVE DEVELOP AIDS
RELATIVELY QUICKLY AND DIE, OTHERS LIVE FOR MANY
YEARS WITHOUT PROGRESSION, OR WITH ONLY SLOW
PROGRESSION TO THE DISEASE. WHY?

HIV DOES NOT NECESSARILY MEAN AIDS

In the early 1980s, after AIDS was recognized but before the discovery of HIV, the disease was regarded as inevitably fatal within a few years. Subsequent studies have shown that while about half of HIV-infected people develop AIDS within ten years, another 25 percent have symptoms suggesting slow progression of the disease, 15 percent experience minor symptoms and test abnormal for immune functions, but up to 10 percent are nonprogressors, living twenty or more years without developing any AIDS-related symptoms or having any laboratory evidence of progression to AIDS.[1] Are nonprogressors real, in the sense that they will never get the disease, or simply extremely slow progressors who will eventually succumb? There are studies to support both possibilities.

FACTORS AFFECTING DISEASE PROGRESSION

It is difficult to find a consensus in the AIDS literature on what factors cause progression or nonprogression from infection to disease, but it is generally thought that the answer to this question may help find containment or cure of AIDS. The mode of transmission of AIDS—whether by sexual contact, intravenous drug use, or through contaminated blood products by transfusion—appears to affect the course of the disease in some studies, but not in others.

Weak mutant strains of the virus have been suggested as a cause of nonprogression or slow progression, and more virulent strains as a cause of rapid progression to AIDS, but this has not been borne out by much of the evidence.

Another factor, which many claim to be crucial in fighting AIDS, is a change in lifestyle: when people living with HIV/AIDS (PLWHA for short) take control of their lives, stop high-risk activities such as unsafe sex and intravenous and recreational drug use, engage in an informed and active way with choice of treatments and therapies, and take an optimistic view of life.

Some studies show that the immune system of the individual does play a large role in slowing down or stopping disease progression, but there is uncertainty about which immunologic response correlates with immunity to AIDS (see the chapter "Vaccinating People Against Their Own Genes") and how useful such information could be to rapid progressors.

In 1993, researchers identified a cluster of thirteen inmates who were infected with the same HIV strain in Glenochil Prison in central Scotland. During the following two years, two went on to develop AIDS and another two developed CD4 counts below 200, while the rest have had much slower progression.[2] Variations in the amount of time taken for progression of disease in individuals infected with the same strain, or indeed any strain of HIV infection, may have something to do with immune system genes called human leukocyte antigen, or HLA. HLA molecules orchestrate the activities of T-cells that fight the infection.[3]

A study reporting strong cytotoxic T-cell and weak neutralizing antibody responses in ten HIV-positive people who were nonprogressors and infected for between eleven and fifteen years showed that they maintained stable T-cell counts above 500. Most importantly, nobody in this study had received antiretroviral treatment.[4]

Indeed, one of the greatest bones of contention as to which factors cause disease progression concerns the efficacy of AZT and HAART offered to PLWHA. AZT was one of the earlier antiretroviral drugs and was superseded by HAART in 1996. HAART consists of combinations of two or more types of antiretroviral agents and a protease inhibitor. These extremely toxic drugs designed to assist in the treatment of HIV/AIDS have been increasingly recognized by many people as a factor in rapid progression to AIDS, with debilitating side effects greatly decreasing the patient's quality of life (see "Anti-HIV Drugs Do More Harm Than Good").

IS AZT/HAART APPROPRIATE TREATMENT FOR PLWHA?

Healthy people who test HIV-positive are assumed to have become infected with HIV. However, antibodies may mean that the virus has been neutralized or put out of action, which may be why infectious HIV is rarely detected in PLWHA.[5]

When faced with an HIV-positive diagnosis, many healthy people have interpreted that as a death sentence and have accepted AZT/HAART as their only hope. But these cytotoxic drugs damage the immune system, which is the body's first line of defense against HIV.

DOES AVOIDING AZT/HAART TREATMENT SLOW OR PREVENT PROGRESSION TO DISEASE?

Some independent scientists, so-called AIDS dissidents, maintain that the number of people newly infected with HIV has been dropping since the 1990s, and that the vast majority of HIV-positive people are long-term survivors, numbering many millions worldwide, including 1 million HIV-positive, healthy Americans and half a million HIV-positive, healthy Europeans. They point out that there is not a single controlled study in the vast AIDS literature proving that HIV-positive people who do not take anti-HIV drugs have a higher morbidity or mortality than HIV-free controls.[6]

Dr. Timothy Hand of Ogelthorpe University in Atlanta, Georgia, and others have documented that long-term survivors abstain from antiviral drugs. He quotes studies suggesting a protective role for cytotoxic CD8-positive T-cells and/or natural killer cells in healthy survivors. These scientists focus on the importance of maintaining cell-mediated immunity, rather than on "killing HIV." They say that HIV infection per se seems to entail little danger, *unless it is followed by antiviral therapy.*

Although many anecdotal reports and numerous scientific studies suggest that most long-term survivors have shunned antiviral drugs, and that the use of antiretrovirals has led to quicker progression to AIDS, Hand maintains these points are often understated in orthodox studies, are not even mentioned in the titles or abstracts, and are sometimes completely overlooked.[7]

Actually, orthodox HIV researchers David Ho and colleagues admitted in one study that no long-term survivors in the study had received antiretroviral therapy. And Alvaro Munoz has reported that not one of the long-term survivors in the largest federally funded study of male homosexuals at risk for AIDS had used AZT.[8]

A study from 1995 showed that fifteen HIV-positive long-term survivors whose CD4 T-cell counts had remained stable for many years had intact immune function and no HIV-related disease. These long-term survivors had taken no antiviral therapy.[9]

Another mainstream HIV study acknowledged that only 38 percent of the healthy long-term HIV-positive subjects had ever used AZT or other nucleoside analogs, compared with 94 percent of those with disease progression.[10]

Dr. Donald I. Abrams, professor of medicine at San Francisco General Hospital and an active participant in AIDS research and treatment from the early 1980s, said at an informal meeting with medical students on October 7, 1996:

> In contrast with many of my colleagues at SFGH in the AIDS program, I am not necessarily a cheerleader for antiretroviral therapy. I have been one of the people who's questioned, from the beginning, whether or not we're really making an impact with HIV drugs and, if we are making an impact, if it's going in the right direction.
>
> I have a large population of people who have chosen not to take any antiretrovirals since I've been following them—since the very beginning. . . . They've watched all of their friends go on the antiviral bandwagon and die, so they've chosen to remain naive [to therapy]. More and more, however, are now succumbing to pressure that protease inhibitors are "it." . . . We are in the middle of the

honeymoon period, and whether or not this is going to be an enduring marriage is unclear to me at this time, so, I'm advising my patients if they still have time, to wait.[11]

Evidence that AZT/HAART is not beneficial to PLWHA has continued to accumulate.

A study reported on ten healthy HIV-positive people in New York City, all of whom had been living with HIV infection for twelve to fifteen years: seven gay men, two intravenous drug users, and one woman infected heterosexually. They had no AIDS symptoms and had normal and stable CD4 cells; they had stopped all high-risk activity after they tested HIV-positive and had no prolonged use of antiretroviral drugs.[12]

In December 1995 the story of Dennis Leoutsakas, Ph.D., was published. He had been HIV-positive for at least seventeen years at the time. He was a former intravenous drug user who had last shared a needle in 1978 and had first tested positive in 1987. With a T-cell count between 650 and 950, Leoutsakas has had none of the opportunistic infections that define AIDS: no pneumonia, Kaposi's sarcoma, or fungal infections. He said that doctors had attempted to explain his case by theorizing that he is infected with a weakened form of HIV. He has never taken AZT or any other antiretroviral drugs.[13] In April 2004, he was appointed to the Advisory Committee on HIV and STD Prevention and Treatment for the Centers for Disease Control, having had at least twenty-six years of nonprogression.[14]

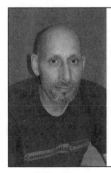

Dr. Dennis Leoutsakas, assistant professor of communication and theater arts at Salisbury University, Maryland, HIV-positive for twenty-six years without progressing to AIDS disease at the time this photo was taken.

The late homosexual AIDS activist Michael Callen found that the overwhelming majority of long-term survivors that he interviewed for his book *Surviving AIDS* had somehow managed to resist the enormous pressure to take AZT, both from a sector of the AIDS community and from medical personnel, and that these survivors had rejected the predominant scientific view that being HIV-positive meant the inevitable decline of the immune system toward an early death. Yet his perception of a person diagnosed with AIDS in 1992 was that "they would sell their grandmother into slavery to get a slot in the latest drug-of-the-month clinical trial."[15]

In contrast, the Toronto Survey on Complementary Therapies found that 78.5 percent of people living with an HIV/AIDS diagnosis used complementary therapies at every stage of illness or recovery and that these people were, on average, more satisfied with every category of complementary therapy than with conventional drugs.[16]

Many researchers as well as PLWHA agree that not only have antiretrovirals not lived up to their promise, they have been a factor in rapid progression to AIDS, causing terrible side effects, such as dementia. However, pharmaceutical companies that have invested large sums of money in the search for these drugs may be an unlikely source of a fresh approach to the understanding of AIDS, and independent researchers have received very little funding or been given very little credibility in the mainstream reporting of AIDS issues. This has led to the suppression of potentially valuable information and the lack of a full and open debate between PLWHA and medical researchers about a more holistic approach to HIV/AIDS.

The fact remains that an unknown number of HIV-positive people throughout the world are surviving and thriving today. The evidence may favor those with a strong natural immunity to HIV who have shunned AZT/HAART and other high-risk activities and who take control of their lives with optimism.

But what about prevention? Would that not solve the problem of becoming infected at all? An effective vaccine against HIV has been the holy grail of the AIDS research establishment from the moment HIV was identified as the "cause" of AIDS. That is just as misguided as the "cure," as we shall see in the next chapters.

The Dangers of
AIDS Vaccine Trials

VACCINE DEVELOPERS AND UNITED NATIONS AGENCIES HAVE
BEEN PUSHING FOR LARGE-SCALE CLINICAL TRIALS OF AIDS VACCINES
IN VULNERABLE THIRD WORLD POPULATIONS RAVAGED BY AIDS.
BUT THERE IS EVIDENCE THAT THE VACCINES ARE
NOT ONLY INEFFECTIVE BUT ALSO DANGEROUS.

NO EFFECTIVE VACCINE IN SIGHT AFTER TWENTY YEARS

The International AIDS Vaccine Initiative (IAVI) describes itself as "a global not-for-profit organization working to accelerate the development of a preventive AIDS vaccine." It was founded in 1996 and operates in twenty-three countries, to "research and develop vaccine candidates." Its major financial supporters include the Bill and Melinda Gates Foundation; the Rockefeller, Sloan, and Starr foundations; the World Bank; Becton, Dickinson & Co.; the European Union; and the governments of Canada, Denmark, Ireland, the Netherlands, Norway, Sweden, the United Kingdom, and the United States.

IAVI published its working-draft paper, "Global Investment and Expenditures on Preventative HIV Vaccines," in July 2004, reaffirming its belief that "the best hope to end the pandemic is a safe and effective preventative HIV vaccine" but admitting that such a vaccine is "still a number of years away."[1]

IAVI also revealed that in 2002, $624 to $670 million was invested in HIV vaccine research and development, with 67 percent coming from the public sector, 17.4 percent from philanthropy, and 15.3 percent from industry. But those figures include the $100 million Challenge Grant awarded to IAVI by the Bill and Melinda Gates Foundation. When that amount is removed, the total investment in 2002 was between $524 and $570 million, of which the public sector accounted for nearly 80 percent, industry for 18 percent, and the philanthropic sector for 2 percent.

As can be seen, vaccine development is big business, with the taxpayer footing 80 percent of the bill. Unfortunately, much of the effort is wasted on vaccines based on a viral gene and its encoded protein, gp120, that are not only ineffective, but could also be dangerous.

THE CULPRIT VIRAL GENE

There is a long list of candidate vaccines against HIV/AIDS, all of them containing gp120, a glycoprotein (protein decorated with side-chains of carbohydrates) belonging to the envelope of HIV-1 (the major class of HIV implicated in AIDS disease). The vaccines include those using re-combinant HIV proteins and peptides (subunit vaccines); others using HIV-1 or SIV (simian immunodeficiency virus, the monkey version of HIV), killed or "attenuated," that is, rendered harmless by successive passage in cultured cells; and a wide range of live recombinant viral, bac-terial, and plasmid vectors expressing (causing the host cell to make) HIV proteins (see box). (Plasmids are pieces of parasitic genetic material exist-ing outside the cell's genome; they are replicated by the cell independently of the cell's genome.)

HIV researcher Dr. Veljko Veljković and his colleagues in Belgrade, Yugoslavia, have been warning against using vaccines containing gp120 since 1990.[2,3] The reason is that the part of the gp120 protein most active in provoking an immune response, the V3 loop and flanking regions, is similar to the antigen-binding region of the human immunoglobulin (Ig) proteins, antibodies produced in an immune response that protect the host against pathogens. Thus, any AIDS vaccine containing the gp120 glycoprotein or the gene coding for it could strongly interfere with the immune system and make the host more vulnerable to the virus. And in the longer term, it could accelerate disease progression in HIV patients who do not yet have symptoms.

The gp120 gene has other properties that pose an even greater threat to the vaccinated population. It contains "recombination hotspots" called

Live Recombinant Viral and Bacterial Vector AIDS Vaccines

Viral Vector Vaccines	Bacterial Vector Vaccines
Vaccinia virus	*Escherichia coli*
Canarypox virus	*Salmonella*
Fowlpox virus	*Shigella*
Influenza virus	*Mycobacterium bovis* BCG
Polio virus	*Streptococcus gordonii*
Venezuelan equine encephalitis virus	*Listeria monocytogenes*
Rabies virus	
Adenovirus	
Hepatitis B virus	
Herpes simplex	
Epstein-Barr virus	
Coxsackievirus	
Attenuated HIV-1	
Vesicular stomatis virus	

Chi (pronounced "kye") similar to those in bacteria and viruses such as *Hemophilus influenzae*, *Mycobacterium tuberculosis*, hepatitis B virus, and herpes simplex virus, which often co-infect with HIV, and that are also similar to recombination elements found in immunoglobulin genes and oncogenes (genes associated with cancer). Recombination hotspots are breakpoints at which genetic exchange or recombination occurs much more frequently than usual.

In fact, Chi-like sequences have been found in the genomes of many multicellular organisms and are suspected to be involved in gene-conversion events, in which the sequence of one gene converts that of another in the genome.[4] This occurs, for example, within the major histocompatibility complex (MHC), a complex of around 100 genes in vertebrates, including the extremely polymorphic (variable) cell-surface proteins called HLA in humans and H-2 in mice, which provide immunological markers for "self" and are involved in immune response against "nonself," including transplants.

Recombination of HIV with bacteria and viruses would generate new pathogens. Within the human host, recombination with human genes would promote chromosomal rearrangements and formation of abnormal immunoglobulins, thus undermining the immune response.

Dr. Veljković's team, in collaboration with researchers in the United Kingdom, Italy, and the United States, have already found evidence of recombination between gp120 and a gene from *Hemophilus influenzae*.[5] A new subtype of HIV-1 may also have resulted from recombination between HIV-1 and SIV.[6]

The proponents of AIDS vaccination trials argue that the desperate situation precipitated by the AIDS epidemic justifies acceptance of the "small risks" involved. But Veljković and his colleagues have written a monograph documenting the lack of efficacy of the vaccines and the enormous risks involved.[7]

INEFFECTIVE AND DANGEROUS

Already in 1994, the AIDS Research Advisory Committee of the National Institutes of Health (NIH) recommended that phase III clinical trials of gp120 vaccines should not be conducted "at this time and in this country." The reasons, according to Dr. Anthony Fauci, director of NIAID, were that the vaccines were ineffective; and there was a remote chance that the vaccines would compromise the immune system and make the recipient more vulnerable to infection.[8]

The possibility that a vaccinated individual runs a greater risk of developing an established infection, or of progressing to disease more rapidly once infected, was confirmed subsequently.[9] The recombinant gp120 subunit vaccine tested in HIV-negative individuals was ineffective in protecting them against infection. Those who became infected during or after vaccination actually had in their blood sera significant levels of antibodies against the vaccine before they became infected, but those antibodies failed to protect them from infection. On the contrary, the vaccine appeared to have acted as a decoy to fool the immune system into mounting an attack on it, while allowing the HIV itself to slip through the host defense to become established.

Nevertheless, a phase III clinical trial for this vaccine in Thailand was announced in 1999.[10]

LIVE RECOMBINANT VIRAL AND BACTERIAL VACCINES

The safety concerns for the individual are bad enough. But it is the effect on vulnerable populations that really worries Veljković and his colleagues, especially from the live recombinant viral and bacterial vector vaccines (see box).

Many viral and bacterial pathogens are being used as vectors, and a number are currently considered "promising" AIDS vaccines. But they are also promising candidates for generating new infectious agents.

THE *SALMONELLA* VACCINE IN UGANDA

The AIDS vaccine based on live *Salmonella* vector was developed by IAVI in partnership with the U.S.-based Institute of Human Virology (IHV) of the University of Maryland and the Uganda Ministry of Health. The development of the "disarmed" *Salmonella* vector expressing HIV-1 gp120 and gp120-derived peptides was started in the early 1990s.

The *Salmonella* vector expressing HIV envelope proteins had been tested in thirty-seven people in a phase I trial by NIAID. Uganda will be the first country in Africa to host a clinical trial of this vaccine.

The only safety concern, it seems, was to ensure that the vaccine did not induce *Salmonella* disease (i.e., diarrhea) in participants;[11] whereas, as Veljković stresses, the right safety question should be: Is the probability for transfer of HIV's genetic material from recombinant *Salmonella* vector to other pathogens equal to zero? To which the answer is an emphatic no. *Salmonella* has the same kinds of Chi recombination hotspots present in gp120, and it is known to exchange blocks of genes with *Escherichia coli* and other bacteria. The potential is rife for generating new pathogens by recombination between the *Salmonella* vaccine and diverse endemic infectious bacteria in Africa.

THE VENEZUELAN EQUINE ENCEPHALITIS
VACCINE IN SOUTH AFRICA

An AIDS vaccine based on the live Venezuelan equine encephalitis (VEE) virus vector, developed jointly by South Africa and the United States,[12] was approved for phase I clinical trials in June 2003.[13] The VEE vaccine was developed by the University of North Carolina at Chapel Hill with five-year federal funding from NIAID totaling more than $12 million.

The stated advantages of the VEE vaccine, according to the developers, are that it targets cells in the lymph nodes, and that "unlike vaccinia virus, poliovirus, adenovirus, herpes viruses and influenza virus-based vaccine vectors, most of the human population have never been exposed to VEE. Therefore immunization to HIV with a VEE-based vector would not be restricted by preexisting immunity to the vector itself."[14] Unfortunately, that is not the case.

VEE virus is carried by arthropods, and it is endemic in northern South America, Trinidad, Central America, Mexico, and Florida; eight different VEE strains have been associated with human disease. These agents also cause disease in horses, mules, burros, and donkeys. Natural infections are acquired by bites from a wide variety of mosquitoes. The same virus was also developed as a biological weapon by the United States in the 1950s and 1960s.

A HERPES SIMPLEX VIRAL VACCINE THAT SHOWS
PROMISE IN NONHUMAN PRIMATES

A modified herpes simplex virus (HSV) that invades host cells and expresses protein from SIV similar to the HIV protein was developed by researchers at Harvard University into a live attenuated AIDS vaccine, which was tested in nonhuman primates. The researchers claim, "HSV vectors show great promise for being able to elicit persistent immune responses and to provide durable protection against AIDS."[15] The same research team has also developed an HSV-2 vector based on another herpes virus, one that is responsible for genital herpes, with the expectation that this vector could serve a double role as a vaccine for HIV as well as for genital herpes.

Unfortunately, the HSV genome contains the greatest number of Chi recombination hotspots of all the microorganisms listed. It also contains Ig class-switch sequences (also recombination hotspots) and other sequences involved in the genetic rearrangements that take place in producing human immunoglobulin genes in blood cells. High levels of recombination have already been identified in the HSV genome associated with these hotspots.

A VACCINIA VIRUS VACCINE LED TO DISEASE AND DEATH

Among the first AIDS vaccines with live viral vectors to be tested in humans was a recombinant, highly attenuated (reduced virulence) vaccinia virus expressing HIV-1 proteins. The vaccinia-gp160 vaccine was developed by Bristol-Myers Squibb, which performed the preclinical study in the period 1985–1988. (The protein gp160 is a precursor of gp120.) The phase I/II research began in 1988 and was dropped in 1993, then continued for an additional year.

These studies combined the vaccinia-gp160 vaccine with a gp160 or gp120 vaccine developed by MicroGeneSys, Chiron, Genentech, and Immuno AG. Unfortunately, a recombinant HIV-vaccine virus arose from the attenuated live vaccine, which was harmful to immune-compromised individuals, producing symptoms of progressive vaccinia (a serious, potentially fatal disease caused by the vaccinia virus) and death.[16] There was also a danger that the recombinant virus could spread and harm other persons with AIDS.

A CANARYPOX VACCINE IN UGANDA, HAITI, TRINIDAD, AND BRAZIL

Another pox virus, the canarypox virus, has been used to create a vaccine. When the canarypox virus carrying HIV genes infects human cells, the cells make proteins from the genes and package them into HIV-like particles called pseudovirions that are noninfectious. These trigger the host immune response against HIV. The first such canarypox viral vaccine carrying the HIV-1 gp160 gene was developed by Pasteur-Mérieux-Connaught;

in combination with Chiron's gp120 construct, it entered a phase II trial in the United States in 1997.

The first phase I trial of a canarypox vaccine in Africa was launched early in 1999. It was tested for safety and immunogenicity (the ability to provoke immune reaction) in Ugandan volunteers, and to reveal the extent to which immunized Ugandans have cytotoxic lymphocytes that are active against the subtypes A and D of HIV, which are prevalent in Uganda. Phase II trials have been completed in Uganda and Brazil. Phase III trials have been planned for several Caribbean countries, Haiti, Trinidad, and Tobago, and Brazil, among other countries. But no phase III trial on this vaccine has so far appeared in the IAVI database.[17]

Is canarypox virus safer than vaccinia virus? Most probably not. Both are orthopox viruses (the same family as the smallpox virus) and are rich in recombination hotspots. This family of viruses is widely distributed, and recombination between different pox viruses can readily take place. Recombinants have arisen that are more virulent than either parent, and it is impossible to predict the fate of released canarypox vaccine with HIV genes. The use of these vaccines in Africa where monkeypox is endemic is likely to generate recombinants with unpredictable potential to cause disease.[18] Monkeypox is transmitted from human to human, but the natural virus is relatively harmless. Could a recombinant virus arise that may be as virulent as the smallpox virus?

AIDS VACCINES FROM PLANTS COULD GENERATE RECOMBINANT VIRUSES THAT SWITCH HOSTS FROM PLANT TO ANIMAL

Finally, AIDS vaccines based on HIV antigens produced in plants are also being developed. The tobacco mosaic virus has been used as a vector to express recombinant coat protein of alfalfa mosaic virus containing antigenic peptides from the rabies virus and HIV-gp120.[19] More recently, Prodigene, a company in Texas, has put gp120 into genetically engineered maize as a cheap, edible oral vaccine against HIV.[20]

There have already been many examples of recombination between viral coat proteins in genetically engineered plants (plants with foreign genetic material inserted into their genomes) and infecting viruses.[21] In addition, there is also evidence that a plant virus has switched hosts to infect vertebrates and recombined with a vertebrate virus.[22]

VACCINE TRIALS IN BREACH OF UNAIDS ETHICAL, SCIENTIFIC, AND SAFETY STANDARDS

According to the 2000 WHO report, more than 90 percent of all AIDS cases are in developing countries. UNAIDS and NIH are the two most important organizations involved in developing AIDS vaccines. UNAIDS executive director Peter Piot has declared, "It is our collective responsibility to ensure that all vaccine trials are conducted under the strictest possible ethical and scientific standards."[23] But Veljković has shown that current vaccines based on HIV-1 gp120 can harm the immune system of individuals and, on account of its recombinogenic tendencies, has the potential to generate deadly viruses and bacteria that can spread through the vaccinated populations and to wildlife. The intended vaccine trials are in serious breach of ethical, scientific, and safety standards.

In the next chapter we shall look at some high-profile failures of "promising" AIDS vaccines.

AIDS Vaccines,
or Slow Bioweapons?

A LONG STRING OF FAILURES IN DEVELOPING VACCINES IS CONFIRMING
THE PREDICTION THAT THESE VACCINES MAY BE WORSE THAN USELESS.

PHASE III VACCINE TRIAL CANCELED

In March 2002, the U.S. government abandoned a controversial AIDS
vaccine trial and announced it would combine the work of two federal
institutions, NIH and the Department of Defense. Both institutions had
proposed trials to test a combination of similar vaccines—a dose of
canarypox virus engineered to carry HIV-1 proteins with a booster shot
of the HIV protein gp120.[1] The trial was designed to compare the types
of immune responses the vaccine evoked with the protection it provided. For the vaccine to pass the trial, it would have to produce an
immune response in at least 30 percent of volunteers. But analysis of the
data showed that the response did not come up to scratch. "It didn't
even come very close," said Dr. Anthony Fauci, director of NIAID. The
canceled NIH trial, which would have involved 11,000 volunteers, was
anticipated to cost $60 to $80 million. The Department of Defense trial,
which was designed to test only the efficacy of the vaccine, will still go
ahead. But that's a grave mistake.

The canarypox vaccine was Aventis Pasteur's ALVAC-HIV (vDP1452),
and the booster, VaxGen's AIDSVAX B/B. The ALVAC vector failed to
provoke a strong immune reaction, and evidence from Dr. Harriet Rob-
inson's team at Emory University, first announced at the Ninth Conference on Retroviruses and Opportunistic Infections (Seattle, Washington,
February 24–28, 2002), demonstrated that adding a gp120 booster to

another vaccine actually reduced the vaccine's efficacy rather than improving it.[2] These disappointing results were as expected, according to AIDS virologists who have been studying the problems of AIDS vaccines for years[3] (see previous chapter).

VACCINES THAT FAIL TO BLOCK INFECTION CAN INCREASE DEATH RATES

More bad news came from vaccine trials in nonhuman primates. Vaccines that induce only cellular immunity through cytotoxic lymphocytes (CTL)—immune cells that destroy cells infected with virus—without circulating antibodies in the plasma gave only partial protection. In a study carried out by researchers in the Merck Research Laboratories in Pennsylvania, Duke University, and Harvard Medical School, two out of fifteen immunized macaque monkeys became ill with AIDS-related symptoms six months after being challenged with the pathogenic HIV-SIV hybrid virus (SHIV).[4]

The best vaccine, based on an adenovirus (a group of viruses that cause respiratory and eye infections) vector, "greatly attenuated" viral infection but did not prevent it. Despite that, the authors claim that the vector was "promising" for development of an HIV-1 vaccine, although they admitted that the relevance of their model system to human HIV-1 infection is not "firmly established" and "cannot be extrapolated to predict human immunogenicity or efficacy." This assessment must be done in clinical trials, they stated.[5] The SHIV hybrid virus, routinely used in such studies, is an especially virulent form of the AIDS virus that kills victims in weeks, and its safety has been strongly questioned.[6]

Another study by researchers based at Harvard Medical School, Northwestern University of Chicago, Duke University Medical Center, and the Southern Research Institute in Maryland was less optimistic.[7] One out of eight immunized rhesus monkeys died as the challenge virus mutated and escaped from the CTL. *Such mutations in the virus that escape immune recognition have been described in more than a dozen reports in the literature in trials involving both humans and nonhuman primates.* The authors concluded, "These data indicate that viral escape from CTL recognition may be a major limitation of the CTL-based AIDS vaccines that are likely to be administered to large human populations over the next several years." This indicates serious safety implications for human vaccines not mentioned by the authors.

As explained in the previous chapter, the vaccines are ineffective and may be harmful to the individuals vaccinated as well as to the populations undergoing clinical trials, by interfering with and undermining the host's immune system and by recombining with viruses and bacteria to generate new infectious pathogens.

A theoretical study by researchers in the Institute of Cell, Animal and Population Biology, University of Edinburgh, Scotland, adds further fuel to the warning. Partially effective vaccines that inhibit the growth of the pathogen but do not prevent infection—*as is the case with most of the AIDS vaccines*—leave death rates unchanged, or worse, increase virulence of the pathogen and deaths as the level of vaccination goes up.[8]

RELEASE OF SLOW BIOWEAPONS IN PHARM CROPS

As mentioned in the previous chapter, a company in Texas, Prodigene, has put gp120 into genetically engineered maize as a cheap, edible oral vaccine against HIV.[9] Veljković and Ho pointed to the potential of widespread contamination of our food crops with disastrous consequences.[10] Based on what is already known concerning the gene and its protein, it is tantamount to releasing a "slow bioweapon" into the population. Not only is this extremely hazardous for human beings, it will affect all organisms in the food chain and multiply the opportunities for the gene to recombine with bacteria and viruses in the environment, of which 99 percent cannot be cultured and are hence completely unknown.

There is now an even more dangerous oral HIV/hepatitis B virus (HBV) combined vaccine, developed in the tomato, with an artificial protein consisting of the env and gag antigens from HIV fused with the HBV major antigenic protein HbsAg.[11] It was publicized in a press release from the Vector State Scientific Center for Virology and Biotechnology in Novosibirsk—the key institution for bioweapons in Russia—as a "pleasant and harmless vaccine," produced jointly with a number of other Russian institutions plus "scientists from the Department for Agricultural Research, Maryland, U.S.A."[12] An article in the *New York Daily News* identified one of the U.S. scientists as Charles Arntzen, founder of the Biodesign Institute at Arizona State University.[13]

AIDS VACCINE WORSE THAN USELESS

The only AIDS vaccine to have progressed past phase III trials, made by VaxGen, took five years and involved 5,108 gay men and 309 women.[14] Unfortunately, it proved ineffective, and may even be harmful.[15]

In the 3,003 white and Hispanic volunteers who received VaxGen's vaccine, a higher proportion suffered breakthrough infections than in the 1,508 controls: 6 percent versus 5 percent. Although the difference is not statistically significant, it could indicate a dangerous trend, suggesting the possibility that the vaccine may have either disarmed the immune system or recombined with an infecting HIV strain to generate a more virulent one. But the company has failed to release further details on the trial results.

The gp120 protein is strongly immunogenic, which is why it has been widely used in vaccines, in the hope that the body will produce antibodies against the protein and hence protect against the virus. But there have been many worrying signs that it may have just the opposite effect.[16] For although the body mounts a strong immune reaction against the protein, and produces antibodies against it, those antibodies fail to protect against the virus. One main reason is that the virus is very mutable and can readily mutate to escape immune detection. In addition, the immune reaction mounted against the original gp120 *undermines* the effectiveness of the immune system by overstimulating it, so that it is less effective to cope with new infections. Indeed, there is emerging evidence that AIDS disease involves an overstimulated, exhausted immune system (see the chapters "Vaccinating People Against Their Own Genes" and "Eating Well for Health").

A recombinant gp120 vaccine tested in HIV-negative individuals in phase I/II trials was not effective in protecting against the disease.[17,18] Not only that, participants in the trials had significant levels of circulating antibodies against the vaccine before they became infected, and they came down with AIDS disease.

The vaccine could thus be dangerous to the vaccinated individual. A vaccine based on the gp120 from the strain SF2 actually suppressed the production of antibodies that could neutralize the later infecting virus, while boosting the production of useless antibodies that were specific for the vaccine strain, SF2.[19] In other words, gp120 appeared to act as a molecular decoy to disarm the body's antiviral response, leaving it more vulnerable and increasing the likelihood of rapid disease progression in those vaccinated who later became infected. This phenomenon is called "deceptive imprinting" of the immune system.[20]

THESE HARMFUL EFFECTS WERE PREDICTABLE AND PREDICTED

Were those effects predictable in advance of the clinical trials? Veljković and his colleagues answer a definite yes.[21]

First, the part of the gp120 molecule that plays the dominant role in provoking an immune response is the V3 loop. The V3 loop and flanking regions are similar in base sequence and structure to the antigen-binding region of the human immunoglobulin (Ig) (antibody protein). And it has been proposed since the early 1990s that this immunoglobulin-like domain in gp120 may interfere with the immune regulatory network.[22] This is strongly supported by later observations that the anti-V3 and anti-Ig antibodies of healthy individuals are similar in structure,[23] and that antibodies reacting to V3 are present in sera that are HIV-negative.[24]

In fact, warnings against AIDS vaccines go back to Albert Sabin, one of the most prominent viral vaccine developers of the twentieth century. "The available data provide no basis for testing any HIV vaccine in human beings either before or after infection," Sabin stated.[25]

An article published in 2003 evaluating the long-term safety of a range of AIDS vaccines involving 3,189 HIV-uninfected, healthy volunteers who were enrolled into fifty-one NIAID-sponsored phase I and II clinical trials concluded that there were no adverse effects.[26] But Veljković remarked, "This conclusion was based on analysis of many important parameters. . . . Unfortunately, the key information—comparison of the health status between breakthrough infected vaccinated volunteers and control subjects who participated in these trials—was not reported, just as it was not reported by VaxGen in the results of their Phase III clinical trial."[27]

Unless this information is reported, said Veljković, the companies and institutions that organized these clinical trials are in danger of committing scientific and ethical misconduct.

Veljković and his colleagues have repeated their call for an immediate moratorium on the clinical trials of HIV-1 gp120/160 vaccines. It appears that their message is finally getting through (see next chapter).

Controversy Breaks over AIDS Vaccine Trials

WITH MANY THOUSANDS OF VOLUNTEERS ENROLLED IN PHASE III ANTI-HIV VACCINE TRIALS TAKING PLACE AROUND THE WORLD, CONTROVERSY OVER THE UTILITY, SAFETY, AND ETHICS OF SOME OF THESE TRIALS HAS SPLIT THE SCIENTIFIC COMMUNITY.

ROW BREAKS OUT AMONG LEADING AIDS RESEARCHERS

A fierce row broke out among leading AIDS researchers in the Policy Forum pages of the January 16, 2004, issue of the journal *Science*. Dr. Dennis R. Burton of the Scripps Research Institute, La Jolla, California, and seventeen other signatories wrote:

> We have concern about the wisdom of the U.S. government's sponsoring a recently initiated Phase III trial in Thailand of a vaccine made from the live-replicating canarypox vector ALVAC with a boost of monomeric gp 120. . . . We doubt whether these immunogens have any prospect of stimulating immune responses anywhere near adequate for these purposes [the aim of the trial]. . . . Multiple phase I and II clinical trials have revealed that the ALVAC vector is poorly immunogenic. The gp 120 component has now been proven in phase III trials in the United States and Thailand to be completely incapable of preventing or ameliorating HIV-1 infection. . . . Our opinion is that the overall approval process lacked input from independent immunologists and virologists, who could have judged whether the trial was scientifically meritorious. . . . As a whole, the scientific community must do a better job of bringing truly promising vaccine candidates to this stage of development and beyond.[1]

A reply appeared on the letters page from Dr. Robert Belshe of St. Louis University School of Medicine and twelve others on July 9, 2004: "If this trial, which has already enrolled and immunised 3000 volunteers, adds to knowledge about HIV vaccine development and prevents even a fraction of future HIV/AIDS cases, its contribution will be very important. . . . Regardless of the specific vaccine efficacy, the trial still will make a substantial contribution to HIV vaccine research because we can apply what we learn to future vaccine candidates."[2] In other words, the volunteers are being used as guinea pigs to contribute to knowledge about HIV vaccine, and neither the efficacy, nor indeed the safety, is considered an issue!

Dr. Robert Gallo, director of the Institute of Human Virology, University of Maryland Biotechnology Institute, and a signatory of Burton's letter, replied independently. He pointed out that, with a number of vaccine candidates in early clinical trials, and new concepts in pre-clinical development looking promising, the high cost of phase III trials could deprive future vaccines of resources. "Therefore, a scientific process that has the courage to abandon products after disappointing phase II trials is essential," he wrote.[3]

Dr. Howard Urnovitz has gone further, accusing the signatories supporting the phase III trial of vested interests that depend on HIV being accepted as the sole cause of AIDS, and on the continued funding of HIV research. He said, "Calling for the creation of a global AIDS vaccine enterprise in the midst of ongoing and widespread failure, rather than focussing on a cure for AIDS, seems a move to further enshrine the HIV concept, and those vested interests." He also points out that Richard D. Klausner, former director of the National Cancer Institute (NCI)—from which the letter in support of the phase III trial was sent—is being investigated for receipt of personal payments from universities and research institutes to which NCI awarded multimillion-dollar research grants during his tenure as director. Howard calls on Congress to open its eyes and investigate where AIDS money is going.[4]

VACCINES SEEN AS THE BEST HOPE AGAINST THE AIDS PANDEMIC

The perceived success of vaccines in the past to control diseases such as smallpox, poliomyelitis, and tuberculosis has persuaded the scientific community that AIDS too could be defeated by the development of a successful vaccine. Many problems have arisen, however, that suggest to some that a vaccine may never be found.

For example, an immune system "primed" by previous exposure to a vaccine may be more susceptible to infection. For although boosting HIV-specific helper cells is important in mediating the host's immune response, it also gives the virus more factories in which to reproduce and mutate.[5] Others maintain that a vaccine may be possible, for instance, because some children born to HIV-positive mothers seem to be protected; and people who develop the disease slowly, or who develop it after many years, seem to be partly protected by their immune system[6] (see the chapter "Anti-HIV Drugs Do More Harm Than Good").

DEVELOPMENT OF GP120 ANTI-HIV VACCINES

Anti-HIV vaccines containing the gp120 envelope protein from the HIV coat are designed to stimulate the immune system of HIV-positive people. The antibody response will neutralize not only the gp120 protein, but also the real protein found on the HIV coat and in HIV-infected cells. These vaccines are also being tested as preventative measures to protect uninfected people from HIV infection.[7] Some vaccines contain the gp120 protein itself, and others use the genetically engineered, or recombinant, gp120 (rgp120) gene, which enables the protein to be synthesized in the cells of those vaccinated (see "The Dangers of AIDS Vaccine Trials").

Companies such as VaxGen, Pasteur-Mérieux, Chiron, and Biocene continue to develop and test gp120- and rgp120-based vaccines derived from strains of HIV prevalent in different ethnic and geographical populations, in spite of the fact that there is no evidence that they work. Back in 1994, the director of NIAID acknowledged that the vaccines were ineffective. They were all but abandoned, but then were taken up in 1995 by VaxGen (see "AIDS Vaccines, or Slow Bioweapons?").

AIDSmap, a U.K.-based AIDS Web site, says, "The most likely outcome is the abandonment of this approach to an HIV vaccine after more than fifteen years of research."[8]

Nevertheless, companies and U.N. agencies have promoted these same vaccines in phase I, II, and large-scale phase III trials around the world. They are now being tested in developing countries such as

Thailand, South Africa, Uganda, and India, which have very vulnerable populations. This irresponsible approach has caused a furor within the AIDS scientific community.

RISKY GP120 VACCINES IN CLINICAL TRIALS AROUND THE WORLD

The dangers of gp120 and the vaccine vectors have been elaborated in the two previous chapters. The failed phase III clinical trial in Thailand (see below) used a canarypox-based vaccine with an AIDSVAX (rgp120) booster, previously tested in Uganda, Haiti, Trinidad, and Brazil. Pox viruses, such as canarypox, monkeypox, and fowlpox, are rich in recombination hotspots and are widely distributed around the world. Recombination between pox viruses happens naturally, but with recombinant canarypox and HIV released together, unpredictable and virulent pathogenic agents could arise.

South Africa is hosting a phase III trial using a vaccine based on the live Venezuelan equine encephalitis (VEE) virus vector expressing rgp120 proteins, developed by South Africa and the United States. As the VEE virus is endemic in South America and elsewhere, it was thought that immunization to HIV with this vector in South Africa would not be restricted by preexisting immunity to the vector itself. It is well known, however, that VEE strains are associated with disease in humans and livestock and are spread by mosquito bite.

A vaccinia virus is also being used in HIV vaccines around the world. In previous studies using the vaccinia vaccine, a recombinant HIV-vaccine virus arose from the live attenuated virus that was harmful to immune-compromised individuals and led to progressive vaccinia and death. Still phase I trials were due to start in India in late 2003 or early 2004, where 4 million people are reckoned to be HIV-positive. The first vaccine will be modified vaccinia Ankara, a live attenuated vaccine developed by Therion Biologics, a company based in Massachusetts.[9]

A clinical trial began in Switzerland and the United Kingdom in June 2003 using NYVAC, a highly attenuated recombinant vaccinia virus bearing envelope genes of HIV-1 (rgp120), developed by Aventis.[10]

In 2005, a combined vaccine using NYVAC as a booster will be used in a second trial all over Europe on people at high risk of HIV infection. If the vaccine is seen to be effective, EuroVacc will vaccinate large sections of the population in Tanzania, Rwanda, South Africa, China, and Russia.[11]

RESULTS OF THE FIRST PHASE III TRIALS

In February 2003, VaxGen released the results of a phase III AIDS vaccine trial in California, which indicated that the vaccine had offered no benefit at all.

Nevertheless, VaxGen claimed that analysis of a small racial subgroup of thirteen individuals showed 78 percent protection to black trial participants. However, with blacks having, on average, a 20 percent admixture of Caucasian genes, it was thought to be unlikely that there would be a twenty-fold difference in efficacy between blacks and the overall study group.[12] This claim was later assessed independently by NIAID and dismissed.

The results did show an association between levels of antibody response to the vaccine and the risk of HIV infection, implying that immune response to the vaccine is a marker for a natural ability to fend off infection. But this was equally present in the placebo recipients.[13]

In November 2003, VaxGen announced its second phase III trial failure: a canarypox-based vaccine, made by Aventis Pasteur, with an AIDSVAX booster adapted for use in Thailand. In this trial, 2,546 recreational intravenous drug users were randomized to receive either the vaccine or a placebo and followed up for three years. The result showed that 3.1 percent of both the vaccinated and placebo groups became infected with HIV each year.[14]

A further complication in Thailand, where expensive PCR testing is not generally available, is that previously vaccinated people being screened for HIV will test positive, even when negative, and may be discriminated against for this reason.[15]

The initiation of another much larger phase III trial in Thailand using the live-replicating canarypox vaccine ALVAC from Aventis Pasteur and an AIDSVAX rgp120 booster, however, was a step too far for some leading researchers.

WE NEED A VACCINE THAT SERVES THE HIV/AIDS COMMUNITY

The problem goes deeper. Large vaccine companies are powerful enough to have control over setting the agenda for trials. They construct their own scientific rationale for their studies, which may not answer the questions that most need to be asked. They also control the data they generate, so that uncomfortable facts that emerge from research do not receive public scrutiny.

Beyond the vaccines' proven inefficacy, some scientists have pointed to a series of hazards and harmful effects of gp120-based vaccines on those vaccinated, including "deceptive imprinting," which could accelerate disease progression[16] (see "AIDS Vaccines, or Slow Bioweapons?").

Reports of fast breakthrough disease progression among volunteers who participated in clinical trials of gp120-based vaccines support these findings. For example, a healthy volunteer who received six rgp120 immunizations acquired an HIV-1 infection 10 weeks later after one high-risk sexual encounter. In spite of an initial low level of detectable infectious virus, a progressive CD4-positive cell decline and dysfunction followed within two years.[17] This may be related to the phenomenon of HIV-positive individuals deteriorating rapidly through acquiring a "superinfection" by another strain of HIV (see next chapter).

While the large, predictably useless, and potentially dangerous phase III trial continues in Thailand, a more encouraging initiative is taking place in that country. An oral therapeutic AIDS vaccine called V-1 Immunitor (V1), comprising pooled HIV antigens, is continuing to show great promise. Recent V1 studies showed body-weight gain, increase in CD4 and CD8 cells, decrease in viral load, and improved survival of end-stage AIDS patients.

The oral vaccine targets mucosal immunity, rather than systemic im-munity, as in injectable vaccines. It is cheap, easy to take, has broad-spectrum activity against many HIV sub-types, and does not require refrigeration. In fact, clinical trials are already proceeding in Africa, with several countries applying for licenses (see "The 'Pink Panacea': An AIDS Vaccine?").

The families and friends of the Thai researchers responsible for V1 paid for its development costs. The researchers remain circumspect about the future of V1; however, in spite of its clinical success as a therapeutic vaccine in over 60,000 HIV-positive patients, in more than fifty countries: "Debates are still being pursued," they said, "as to what is the best strategy for developing a potent AIDS vaccine. Despite our advances in modern technology we may have failed to appreciate and take into account the simple fact that retroviruses are unlike other viruses and that a radically different, perhaps counterintuitive immunological approach might be required."[18]

The ethos of this enterprise could not be in sharper contrast to that of the mainstream vaccine research community, which is currently asking for more public funding to develop a vaccine similar to those that have failed so badly for so long. The consequences of AIDS research following the money instead of the cure are now compounding health and environmental problems around the world, as well as wasting billions of dollars.

Vaccinating People Against Their Own Genes

COMPLEXITIES IN THE IMMUNE RESPONSE ARE FRUSTRATING
ALL CURRENT ATTEMPTS AT CREATING EFFECTIVE VACCINES,
AND MAY END UP VACCINATING PEOPLE AGAINST THEIR OWN GENES.

THE BODY'S DEFENSE SYSTEM

Immunity is the body's defense against foreign agents and diseased cells. It includes physical, chemical, and microbiological barriers such as the skin and mucous membranes, as well as a network of lymphoid organs, tissues, cells, "humoral" factors circulating in bodily fluids, and cytokines (proteins secreted by immune cells that affect the function of other cells).

There are two components to immunity: innate and acquired (or adaptive), although they are not at all separate from each other.

Innate immunity includes the physical, chemical, and microbiological barriers, but more usually refers to the immune system, consisting of several classes of white blood cells—complement, cytokines, and acute phase proteins—which provide the immediate line of host defense. It is rapid and nonspecific and may end up damaging normal tissues if unbalanced.

Adaptive immunity consists of antigen-specific reactions through other classes of white blood cells, the T- and B-cells. It is precise, but it takes several days or weeks to develop; furthermore, it has memory, so subsequent exposure to the same antigen leads to a more vigorous and rapid response.

INNATE IMMUNITY

The main feature of innate immunity is the recruitment and activation of white blood cells called *neutrophils* at the site of infection. The same process occurring inappropriately leads to inflammatory connective tissue disease and the systemic inflammatory response syndrome. *Neutrophils*—defined by their staining properties—are recruited by *macrophages*, large white blood cells that phagocytose (engulf) the infecting agent and send out several chemical signals referred to as cytokines.

Cytokines are a diverse group of proteins and peptides secreted by immune cells to alter their own behavior or that of other cells. Two cytokines—granulocyte-stimulating factor and granulocyte-macrophage colony-stimulating factor—produced by macrophages stimulate division of specific cells in the bone marrow, resulting in the release of millions of neutrophils into circulation, which become attracted to the site of infection. There, they engulf the infecting agents, killing them by producing toxic oxygen products such as hydrogen peroxide, or toxic proteins and enzymes. Ingestion and killing of microorganisms are 100 times more effective if they have been decorated with specific antibody, or "complement."

The *complement* system consists of at least twenty serum proteins activated in a cascade, so that activating a single molecule generates thousands of effector molecules. These effector molecules eventually bind to the protective membrane of the virus or bacterium, making holes through the membrane, thereby killing the virus or bacterium.

Natural killer cells recognize abnormal or infected cells and kill them, in two ways. First, they have immunoglobulin receptors that recognize targets coated with antibodies. Second, they have receptors on their surface for major histocompatibility complex (MHC) class I proteins that define "self." If these receptors don't find MHC on the target cell, the natural killer cell will destroy the target cell.

Although not antigen-specific, the innate system can discriminate foreign molecules from self and enable eradication of infectious agents such as bacteria. It is not able, however, to detect intracellular agents, notably viruses.

ADAPTIVE IMMUNITY

Adaptive immunity starts when the macrophage engulfs the infective agent, such as a virus, breaks it down, and displays bits of the virus (antigens) on its cell surface. This signals the helper T-cells, each of which carries a different receptor on its cell surface, to bind to the antigen; but only the T-cell with a receptor that fits the antigen displayed on the macrophage will bind to it. This binding stimulates the macrophage to produce cytokines such as interleukin-1, which in turn stimulates the helper T-cell to produce other cytokines, interleukin-2 and interferon-γ. Interleukin-2 instructs other T-cells to multiply, resulting in the release of two classes of effector T-cells: CD4 helper T-cells, and CD8 cytotoxic T-cells.

The CD4 cells come in two subclasses, T-helper cells 1 and T-helper cells 2 (Th1 and Th2). Th1 cells produce interleukin-2, which induces T-cell proliferation and stimulates CD8 T-cell division and cytotoxicity, and interferon-γ, which activates macrophages to kill intracellular pathogens such as mycobacteria, fungi, and protozoa, and induces natural killer cells to cytotoxicity. This is the type 1 or cell-mediated immune response. Interleukin-12 is secreted by the interferon-γ-stimulated macrophages, which further increases interferon-γ production by T-cells. Th1 response is inflammatory and contributes to autoimmune diseases.

Th2 CD4 cells produce interleukins-4, -5, -6, and -10, which favor antibody production in the type 2 or humoral immune response. They cause B-cells to multiply and secrete antibodies to circulate in the body fluids. Interleukin-4 provides positive feedback to induce further Th2 response and is associated with allergic disease.

B-cells produce antibodies, which serve to neutralize toxins and prevent organisms from adhering to mucosal surfaces. The antibodies released by the B-cells bind to antigens on the surface of free viruses, making it easier for macrophages to destroy them, and also signal blood components called complement to puncture holes in the viruses. B-cells can respond to antigens independently of T-cells or with the help of T-cells.

Different classes of antibodies predominate in different compartments of the body. For example, IgG is the main class of antibodies in the blood and other tissues, whereas IgA is in secretions of the mucosa.

As infection is brought under control, the activated T- and B-cells are turned off by suppressor T-cells. A few memory B- and T-cells remain behind to respond quickly if the same virus attacks again.

B- and T-cells are both lymphocytes produced in the bone marrow. If they mature within the bone marrow, they are referred to as B-cells; if in the thymus gland, T-cells. The bone marrow and the thymus are known as primary lymphoid organs. Organized lymphoid tissue elsewhere is known as secondary lymphoid tissue and includes the lymph nodes, adenoids, tonsils, and mucosa-associated lymphoid tissues (MALTs). MALTs are present in the bronchus, the gut, the nasopharynx, and the urogenital system. These lymphoid organs receive antigens from the tissues and mucosal surfaces. Antigens that succeed in getting into the bloodstream are intercepted in the spleen.

The production of antigen-specific receptors and antibodies in both T-cells and B-cells results from a remarkable process of DNA rearrangement and splicing together of multiple separate segments coding for the antigen-binding regions of the immunoglobulins. This occurs early in the development of the cells, before exposure to antigen. Each cell and its descendants (which form a clone) eventually end up expressing only one immunoglobulin or receptor. This produces a repertoire of 108 T-cell receptors and 1010 antibody specificities in the T- and B-cell populations, adequate to cover the range of pathogens that the body is likely to encounter.

DELICATE BALANCE OF A VERY COMPLEX SYSTEM

The above is an extremely simplified outline of a very complex immune system,[1-3] the different components of which have to be delicately balanced to work effectively in defending the host, while not harming the host itself. Thus, attempts to change one component invariably result in affecting several others. Individual cytokines, for example, tend to have different effects on different cells depending on the concentrations of other cytokines present. High concentrations of the cytokine will commonly cause shedding of the corresponding receptors from cell surfaces, thereby reducing further responses.

The immune system works in close communication with other tissues; especially well documented is the interaction of immune cells with the neurological and endocrine systems.

THE MIND–BODY CONNECTION

The immune system and the nervous system are connected anatomically and functionally.[4] The lymphoid organs are richly supplied with nerves; and neurotransmitters such as acetylcholine, norepinephrine, and vasoactive intestinal peptide (see the chapter "Exercise Versus AIDS") are released at nerve endings to modulate immune activity. Receptors for these neurotransmitters are present on lymphocytes, as are receptors for neuroendocrine hormones such as corticotropin-releasing factor (CRF), leptin, and α-melanocyte-stimulating hormone (MSH), which are essential for regulating cytokine balance and the inflammatory response.

CRF is released from the hypothalamus in response to environmental stress and activates the pituitary to produce adrenocorticotropin hormone (ACTH), which in turn activates the adrenal glands to produce corticosteroids. Increased CRF inhibits Th1 immunity and the inflammatory response. Leptin, produced in response to levels of fat stores, regulates body weight and is a potent stimulator of Th1 immunity. MSH, in contrast, inhibits activation of transcription factors and is anti-inflammatory. The immune system modulates brain activity, including body temperature, sleep, and feeding behavior, through various cytokines that pass through the blood–brain barrier. Molecules such as the MHC not only direct T-cells to immunogenic molecules but are also involved in the development of normal connections between neurons in the brain and in neurological memory.

It has been possible to demonstrate modulation of the immune response with behavioral experiments in which stressed animals show activation of CRF and adrenocorticoids, which suppress immune response. Similarly, classical behavioral modification techniques can produce immune suppression. Operant conditioning, in which a behavioral outcome is paired with a positive or negative stimulus, has been used to train lupus-prone mice to successfully suppress manifestations of autoimmunity.

Psychoimmunology, the physical influence of mind/feeling on the immune system, is now an established discipline that has compelled even the most reductionist scientists to adopt a more holistic perspective on health. It is not surprising, therefore, that long-term HIV survival is associated with the ability of individuals to take control of their own lives with optimism, an association that needs to be much more extensively researched than it has been (see "Surviving and Thriving with HIV").

HOW THE NATURAL IMMUNE RESPONSE
MAY ACT AGAINST HIV INFECTION

There appear to be at least three immune reactions to HIV antigens in high-risk subjects who nonetheless remain seronegative: cell-mediated immune reactivity (CMI), antibodies in mucosal secretions, and (false-) positive reaction in the urine but not in the serum,[5] owing to autoantibodies against endogenous viral proteins that cross-react with the HIV antigens (see "HIV and Latent Viruses").

CMI reactivity to HIV-1 antigens in seronegative subjects is well documented. For example, HIV-1–specific T-cell reactivity to *env* antigens was detected in seronegative healthcare workers exposed to HIV-1–contaminated blood.[6] Pinto and co-workers reported *env*-specific (gp160) cytotoxic T-cell reactivity in seronegative subjects who had been exposed to accidental needlesticks contaminated with HIV-1–positive blood;[7] they cited ten further publications reporting CMI responses to HIV-1 antigens in high-risk seronegative subjects.

Mazzoli and co-authors reported both the occurrence of CMI in serum and IgA (reactivity to an HIV-1 gp160) in urine and vaginal wash specimens obtained from seronegative sexual partners who were HIV-1 positive.[8]

Another kind of cell-mediated immunity was specific cytotoxic T-cell reactivity to the HIV-1 antigens *nef, pol*, and p24 and p17 peptides found in six seronegative commercial sex workers in Gambia, West Africa.[9] The strongest responses were to *pol* and *nef*.

A revealing study involved three cohorts of Kenyan women: HIV-1–resistant commercial sex workers, HIV-1–infected commercial sex workers, and low-risk women. Resistance was defined as persistent seronegativity to HIV-1 antigens and negative reverse transcription PCR assays for HIV-1 sequences for three or more years of commercial sex work.

Cervicovaginal washes from all subjects were tested for HIV-1–specific IgA and IgG. T-helper lymphocyte response (CMI) to HIV-1 antigens was also determined. HIV-1–specific IgA was present in sixteen of twenty-one HIV-1–resistant commercial sex workers (76 percent), five of nineteen HIV-infected commercial sex workers (26 percent), and three of twenty-eight low-risk women (11 percent). CMI was present in eleven of twenty-five resistant women (55 percent), four of eighteen HIV-infected women (22.2 percent), and one of twenty-five low-risk women (4 percent). The authors suggest that a protective mucosal immune response to HIV-1 infection can operate independently of CMI response.[10]

Considered together, the findings document an important role of natural CMI and mucosal immunity mediated by IgA in resistance to HIV-1 infection. Thus inappropriate immunizations can destroy or interfere with this natural immunity, and worse.

FURTHER COMPLICATIONS

Broadly speaking, there are three types of HIV infections: monotypic, in which a single subtype causes infection; multitypic, in which more than one subtype causes infection; and infections by "mosaics" that are recombinants between or among single subtypes. All these are known to occur in humans and in the individual tissue compartments such as the gut, the reproductive system, the blood, and the brain. Moreover, mosaic subtypes generated in a given tissue compartment are known to differ from those in a different tissue compartment *in the same host.*

Thus, cloned sequences of viral populations derived from semen and peripheral blood mononuclear cells were different;[11] so were HIV-1 strains derived from the blood and genital compartments. Analysis of *env* gene sequences (V1, V2, and V3) in infected cells obtained from cervical secretions and peripheral blood mononuclear cells (PBMCs) were carried out on six women who had just become HIV-positive.[12] Three patterns of diversity were found: homogeneity between cervical and PBMC-derived strains, variants of cervical and PBMC origin with modest heterogeneity within each genotype, and multiple variants within each compartment.

Epstein and co-workers reported on the tissue-specific evolution (brain and spleen) of HIV-1 variants in children with AIDS, and used the term *quasispecies* to describe HIV-1 variants. They found that brain and spleen HIV-1 populations differed from each other and that each population evolved independently.[13]

A study of Thai subjects in 1995 reported "the first evidence of dual HIV-1 infection of humans by subtypes B and E."[14]

SUPERINFECTION

By 2003, researchers had discovered that "superinfection" with more than one HIV strain was more common than previously thought. Luc Perrin, a professor of clinical virology at the University of Geneva, Switzerland, was following 136 HIV-positive drug users when he found that the viral load of five patients jumped suddenly after years of suppression without treatment. Two of them had become (super-)infected with another HIV strain.[15] Harold Burger of Albany Medical College in New York presented genetic analysis data from an HIV-positive woman in which two HIV strains recombined to produce a new hybrid.[16]

"Superinfection is sobering," Anthony Fauci, director of NIAID, is reported to have said. "That means that, although you can mount an adequate response against one virus, the body still does not have the capability to protect you against new infection, which tells you that the development of a vaccine is going to be even more of a challenge."[17]

A retrospective analysis of primary infection in a cohort of seventy-eight gay men uncovered three cases (5 percent) of superinfection with a second virus.[18] This led to a negative impact on CD4 cell count and viral load six months later. Thus, no protection against the second infection was afforded by the successful immune suppression of the original HIV strain, which was equivalent to a vaccination. Instead, if anything, it made the individuals deteriorate much faster. This phenomenon is reminiscent of the "deceptive imprinting" of the immune system in people given the gp120 vaccine, which made them vulnerable to subsequent infection by HIV (see "AIDS Vaccines, or Slow Bioweapons?").

Genetic diversity and tissue compartmentalization are hallmarks of HIV-1 infection. Thus, a vaccine consisting of a single subtype is most likely to be ineffective, could well be misdirected to the wrong tissue compartment, and could make things worse through deceptive imprinting for HIV-negative individuals; and for those already HIV-positive, vaccinating could create new recombinant strains that escape immune containment.

IMMUNE STATUS OF LONG-TERM SURVIVORS

Researchers at Imperial College, London University, and Westminster Hospital in the United Kingdom carried out a study to compare the immune status of "clinical nonprogressors" with "chronic progressors," "immunologically discordant progressors," and control subjects.[19] *None of the subjects in any category had taken antiviral or other forms of recognized AIDS therapy.*

The ten clinical nonprogressors had been infected with HIV-1 for more than five years and had an undetectable viral load and a stable CD4 T-cell count (median, 824 cells/μl; range, 480 to 1,130 cells/μl). The three immunologically discordant (between T-cell and viral load markers) progressors had been infected with HIV-1 for more than ten years and showed a decline in CD4 T-cell numbers but maintained a low viral load in the absence of antiretroviral treatment. The seventy patients with chronic progressive HIV-1 disease (clinical progressors) had a decreasing CD4 T-cell count (median, 285 cells/μl; range, 86 to 420 cells/μl) and high plasma viral load (median, 165,220 copies/μl; range, 5,492 to more than 500,000 copies/μl).

Blood samples were drawn from all the subjects and from twenty HIV-negative controls, and peripheral blood mononuclear cells were isolated to examine how the cells responded to different challenges.

The researchers found that the cells from clinical progressors lacked T-helper lymphocytes that respond to HIV-1 challenge, either by cell proliferation or by producing cytokines. In contrast, clinical nonprogressors responded to a wide range of HIV-1 antigens from different clades (evolutionary groups or families of variants), producing both Th1 (promoting cell-mediated immune response) and Th2 cytokines (promoting humoral antibody response). Immunologically discordant progressors responded strongly to clade B Gagp24 antigen with a Th1 cytokine profile, but not to other antigens. Neither clinical progressors nor immunologically discordant progressors secreted interleukin-4 in response to HIV-1 antigens. No HIV-1 specific T-cell responses were seen in twenty seronegative controls.

There was a rapid Th1-to-Th2 shift in the response of one immunologically discordant progressor at the onset of clinical symptoms.

The responses of nonprogressors to the majority of other viral antigens were comparable to those seen in uninfected controls. Interestingly, nonprogressors showed significantly increased responses to herpes simplex virus and cytomegalovirus antigens compared to uninfected controls, as found previously, suggesting that they have also successfully defended themselves against infections by those agents (see "HIV and Latent Viruses").

As the authors remark, these results suggest that a balanced Th1/Th2 profile correlates with successful long-term control of HIV-1. Vaccination in such subjects is likely to unbalance their natural immune response and make things worse for them.

The findings also suggest that a therapeutic approach to rebalancing the immune system in chronic progressors and immunologically discordant progressors is preferable to the use of toxic antiviral drugs.

VACCINATING PEOPLE "AGAINST THEIR OWN GENES"

More importantly, evidence is presented in the next chapter that HIV may have arisen as the result of recombination between SIV and human genes; that HIV has the ability to recombine yet further with other human genes; and that it may reactivate latent viruses hiding in the genome.

Thus, vaccinating people against HIV would amount to vaccinating people "against their own genes," as Dr. Howard Urnovitz said in his testimony to the U.S. House of Representatives in 1999, with disastrous consequences, including the potential of autoimmune disease.[20]

But even that is not the whole story.

HIV and Latent Viruses

HIV MAY NOT BE THE CAUSE OF AIDS. THE REAL KILLER
MAY BE RNAS CREATED FROM SCRAMBLED GENOMIC
SEQUENCES OR LATENT VIRUSES THAT ARE REACTIVATED
BY TOXIC DRUGS AND ENVIRONMENTAL AGENTS.

A STRANGE CASE OF AIDS AND GENE SHUFFLING

Back in 1999, Dr. Howard Urnovitz and colleagues identified a mysterious case of AIDS in a French woman with apparently no risk factors as usually defined.[1] The forty-one-year-old was originally diagnosed in 1986 with a low white blood cell count associated with cervical carcinoma, progressed to a depletion of CD4 T-cells with opportunistic infections, and eventually died in 1992. The initial diagnosis of "idiopathic CD4 T-cell lymphocytopenia" (meaning "strange disease with depleted CD4 T-cells") was changed to AIDS when a group O strain of HIV-1, HIV-1vau, was isolated from the patient.

Analysis of the HIV viral envelope from the patient revealed that it appeared to be copied from stretches of DNA present on fourteen different human chromosomes, most of them from chromosome 7, especially the region 7q31. This region of chromosome 7 contains mutations and recombinations linked to several cancers. In addition, a short stretch similar to the African green monkey immunodeficiency virus envelope protein gene was found.

This opened a whole new can of worms. Was this rare strain of HIV-1 the result of genetic recombination (reshuffling) in the human genome? Urnovitz and colleagues had identified similar extensive genetic recombination in veterans suffering from Gulf War syndrome, which they believed to have resulted from exposure to toxic agents in the environment.[2,3] The French woman was a farm worker who could have been exposed to toxic agrochemicals.

HIV: A RECOMBINANT BETWEEN SIV AND HUMAN GENES?

Urnovitz and Murphy had earlier suggested that HIV-1 itself might be a recombinant between the simian immunodeficiency virus (SIV) and human "endogenous retroviral sequences,"[4] which make up some 8 percent of the human genome.[5] SIV capable of causing AIDS in monkeys appears to occur exclusively in African monkeys, particularly in the African green monkey.

One theory proposes that the AIDS virus may have come from early polio vaccines that consisted of the poliovirus propagated in rhesus and African green monkey kidney cells. At least twenty-six monkey viruses, including adenoviruses, cosackievirus, herpesvirus, echovirus, and possibly other groups of viruses, were found as contaminants in such preparations. SIV could be among the contaminants, at least in some batches of the vaccine. If so, SIV could have recombined with endogenous retroviral sequences in people given the vaccine. Urnovitz and Murphy pointed out that DNA sequences related to the highly conserved (almost identical) domain of the HIV reverse transcriptase and glycoprotein gp41 (part of the gp160 polyprotein of HIV-1 that is cleaved into gp120 and gp41) have been found in the human genome.

Given the similarities between HIV and human genome sequences, further recombination is to be expected.

HIV is thought to replicate in a wide variety of tissues; as a retrovirus, it would integrate its genome into the host cell genome, it would have an extraordinarily high mutation/recombination rate, and multiple subtypes could infect a subject at the same time (see "Vaccinating People Against Their Own Genes"). HIV-1 subtypes not only recombine with each other but may also recombine with human retrotransposons (mobile genetic elements similar to retrovirus genomes) or human chromosome segments.[6]

As mentioned in the chapter "AIDS Vaccines, or Slow Bioweapons?" the V3 loop and its flanking regions in the HIV gp120 gene are located between recombination signals similar to those found in human immunoglobulins (as well as in many bacteria and viruses). Consequently, the immunologically dominant region of gp120 may also be involved in recombining with human immunoglobulin genes. This can either disarm the immune response to HIV, or else give rise to auto-immune response, in which the body effectively produces antibodies against its own proteins.

HIV ACTIVATES ENDOGENOUS VIRUSES

Apart from recombining with host genes, HIV-1 infection may activate human endogenous retroelements (including retroviruses and retro-transposons) with or without recombination, simply by expressing gene functions that can help mobilize those elements. In other words, HIV infection can activate latent viruses in the genome, which may themselves have deleterious effects.

For example, a family of human endogenous retrovirus, HERV-K, represented by fifty more or less full-length viral genomes, was found to have a protein, nuclear RNA export factor, that is similar to the HIV-1 Rev protein, carries out the same function, and is interchangeable with it.[7] The researchers suggested that HIV-1 infection might promote HERV-K expression in humans, pointing out that some 70 percent of HIV-1–positive patients were reported to express antibodies recognizing HERV-K structural proteins, whereas little or no reactivity was observed among HIV-1–negative blood donors.

Indeed, Urnovitz's team found antibodies to human endogenous retroviruses in the urine of patients with clinical AIDS, which correlate with the progression of disease.[8] These antibodies tend to cross-react with HIV-1 antigens, yielding false-positives in the urine of HIV-negative people. In his contribution to the AIDS Conference in Durban, South Africa, in 2000, Urnovitz said this finding was the turning point for his thinking about AIDS in a different way.[9]

AIDS A "GENOMICS DISEASE"

"My hypothesis is that AIDS is a genomics disease with an associated virus called HIV," said Urnovitz.

Urnovitz is not even sure that the virus HIV exists. He thinks it may simply be a piece of RNA containing reshuffled gene sequences similar to those found in people exposed to a variety of environmental toxic agents, as in veterans suffering from Gulf War syndrome. In other words, what many scientists have been calling HIV may be a marker for having been exposed to toxic agents that are likely to lead to AIDS disease, but may not be the actual agent that causes the disease. This harks back to Peter Duesberg's idea that AIDS disease is caused by recreational and injected drugs (see the chapter "AIDS and HIV") and that HIV is just an "innocent bystander" virus.

What impressed Urnovitz was the appearance of certain HERV antibodies in the late stages of AIDS disease, which suggested to him that endogenous viral genes (or the viruses) could play a "strong role" in AIDS progression.

ARE HERVS THE CULPRIT?

There are many families of endogenous retroviral-like elements in the human genome, which include both retroviruses and retrotransposons, both of which are capable of multiplying by making RNA copies of themselves that are reverse-transcribed into complementary DNA and integrated into new sites in the genome. The difference between retrotransposons and retroviruses is that the former lacks an envelope. Most HERV families consist of multiple copies of an element, some of which are complete and active, while the rest are defective, but could be mobilized with the help of other elements.

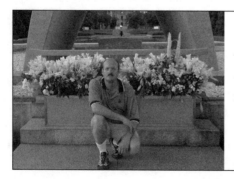

Dr. Howard Urnovitz in Hiroshima.

There is a great deal of evidence that HERV genes are expressed in human cells,[10] although the triggers for gene expression are not completely understood. For example, it is known that inflammatory responses induced by tissue injury, toxic chemical agents, radiation, or infectious agents contribute to activating genes on transposable elements.[11] A particular class of short interspersed elements, called *Alu*, are activated by HIV-1 infection.[12] It appears that the HIV *tat* (transactivating) protein boosts the transcription of *Alu* retrotransposons by increasing the activity of the transcription factor TFIIIC.

Alu elements compose 10 percent of the human genome and are increasingly recognized as "molecular genetic engineers" in the genome. They respond to physiological and environmental signals to move blocks of genetic material around with them and to rejoin them in new configurations.[13] The activation of *Alu* elements and recombination mediated by these elements are contributing factors in the progression of some chronic diseases such as Gulf War syndrome.[14] Urnovitz and co-workers found RNAs circulating in the bloodstream of patients that were derived from scrambled segments in a region of chromosome 22. It is as though something had chopped up that region of chromosome 22 into pieces, shuffled them, and joined them together again, and *Alu* elements appeared to be the culprit.[15] Furthermore, at least some of these sequences are unique to Gulf War syndrome and could be diagnostic of the condition.

INFECTIOUS RNAS ARE NOT VIRUSES

These new species of RNA, *which have no correspondence to actual sequence in the host germline genome*, are enclosed in membranous vesicles and circulating in the bloodstream of patients. They could thus easily be mistaken for RNA viruses or retroviruses.

There are typically numerous RNA sequences circulating in disease states, and at least some of them are associated with the disease. There is evidence that these RNAs are capable of "infecting" the blood cells of healthy animals in a mouse disease-model and transmitting the disease.

Is there a human equivalent? In 1983, the same year that Dr. Luc Montagnier's team reported the discovery of the virus believed to cause AIDS,[16] Dr. Gene Shearer proposed that AIDS is a "graft versus host" disease.[17] In other words, something, not necessarily a virus, was in the semen of men suffering from AIDS that was passed on to a recipient who, in turn, developed the disease. That "something" could have been a reshuffled genome sequence represented in the circulating RNAs.

Urnovitz has since detected unique "nonblueprint" (nongermline genomically encoded) plasma RNAs in other chronic diseases, including mad cow disease, which he claims offers a predictive diagnostic test for the disease in animals before the symptoms appear. The scientific establishment ignored his work for years. But in April 2005, Urnovitz was awarded a grant of up to $650,000 from the German Ministry for Education and Research to develop just such a test.[18]

Urnovitz may well be on the right track, as geneticists have been unearthing more and more of the vast RNA underworld that mediates between DNA and proteins.[19]

RNA INTERFERENCE AND DISEASE

Since Urnovitz discovered nonblueprint circulating RNA sequences, there has been a sea change in how RNA is perceived in molecular biology.

RNA used to be thought of as the molecular "messenger" or go-between that transmits the genetic instruction in DNA to proteins, which are the "bricks" and "workhorses" in the organism. As the human genome was mapped and sequenced, however, it became clear that the proportion of DNA that codes for proteins is only 1.5 percent of the human genome. And 97 to 98 percent of the RNA transcribed from the DNA does not code for proteins. So what is all that extra RNA doing in the organism?

Apparently, this extra RNA "interferes" copiously in the workings of the organism. There is a vast underworld of RNA that appears to be necessary for survival. On the surface, it is like an enormous espionage network in which genetic information is stolen or gets rerouted as it is transmitted, or transformed, corrupted, destroyed, and in some cases, returned to the source file in a totally different form.

The inescapable conclusion is that the job of mediating between DNA and protein is really at the center stage of molecular life. And who gives orders to the multitudes of RNA agents? In a sense it is everyone and no one, because the organism works by perfect *inter*communication of all its parts, not by linear chains of commands that go strictly one way from DNA to RNA to protein. Intercommunication is the essence of the "fluid and dynamic genome" uncovered by genetic engineering techniques since the mid-1970s, which has consigned the old static framework of classical genetics to the dustbin. But that is another story.[20]

The point is that different species of RNA are now known to have key roles in regulating and coordinating gene functions. So it would not be surprising if at least some of Urnovitz's nonblueprint RNA had drastic effects on people's health.

As plausible as Urnovitz's hypothesis seems, he too may not have the entire story on the causes of what has been collectively lumped together as AIDS disease that is blamed on HIV. Yet another connection to a latent virus lurking in the human genome was made in the 1990s.

THE HERPES VIRUS CONNECTION

Dr. Robert Gallo in the United States was credited with the joint discovery of HIV as the cause of AIDS after an acrimonious challenge from the French Pasteur Institute, whose scientist, Dr. Luc Montagnier, in the opinion of the majority of the AIDS research community, had actually identified the correct virus.[21]

Gallo and colleagues were among the first, however, to demonstrate the presence of a human herpes virus, HHV-6, in the vast majority of tissues from AIDS patients, while in contrast, HIV-negative controls had restricted tissue distribution and a significantly lower infection level of HHV-6.[22] There was also a significant correlation between the frequency and extent of HHV-6 infection and the CD4 T-cell count. So is it reasonable to think that HHV-6 may be the real cause of the AIDS disease rather than HIV? No, according to the AIDS research establishment; the HIV-AIDS connection has taken such a firm hold that nothing else is conceivable. Instead, Paolo Lusso and Robert Gallo suggested that HHV-6 acts as an "accelerating factor" for disease progression.

One big problem with HHV-6 is that it is a virus present in some 90 percent of the general population, and there is already a wide spectrum of ailments attributed to it.[23] In immune-suppressed patients, this includes fever, hepatitis, failure of bone marrow engraftment, encephalitis, and interstitial pneumonitis. In immunocompetent adults, HHV-6 has been linked to infectious mononucleosis, autoimmune disorders, chronic fatigue syndrome, fulminant hepatitis, non-Hodgkin's lymphomas, and Hodgkin's disease.

HHV-6 is a member of the herpes virus family and closely related to human cytomegalovirus (CMV). Like other members of this family, it causes a primary infection and then can establish latent infection for the lifetime of the infected host, often by integrating into the genome of the host cells. Some researchers think that the salivary glands are a reservoir and thus the virus can spread via saliva. Others suggest the central nervous system serves as the site for persistent infection. In most individuals, the virus remains quiescent for life; but under immune suppression and other unknown circumstances, such as HIV-1 infection or exposure to environmental toxic agents, the virus can be reactivated.

HHV-6 primarily infects T-lymphocytes and hence has the potential to interact with HIV-1. Some investigators have proposed that HIV-1 directly causes reactivation of HHV-6 in doubly infected cells. Cells doubly infected *in vitro* (in the test tube) showed an increase in HHV-6. HHV-6 also enhances HIV-1 replication by *trans*-activating (activating by a diffusible factor, such as a protein encoded by the virus) the transcription and hence replication of HIV-1, and increases HIV recognition of T-cells by causing the expression of CD4—the receptor for HIV—on T-cells and natural killer cells.

Is HHV-6 more frequent in HIV-positive people? Some researchers used PCR to detect HHV-6 in saliva and found it less frequently in HIV-seropositive patients than in HIV-seronegative patients.[24]

Dr. Konnie Knox and Dr. Donald Carrigan at the Medical College of Wisconsin, Milwaukee, however, used immunohistochemical staining to detect the active virus and found evidence of infection in 100 percent of HIV-positive patients.

HHV-6 INFECTION AND AIDS

Knox and Carrigan examined thirty-four autopsy samples harvested from nine people who had died of AIDS in a Milwaukee hospital. All thirty-four tissue samples of lung, lymph node, liver, kidney, and spleen revealed active HHV-6 infection at the time of death. CMV, by contrast, was present in only nine samples. HHV-6 had in particular attacked the lungs of all nine patients. In one of the six who died from respiratory failure, the density of HHV-6 was so great that the virus appeared to be responsible for killing the patient.[25]

A year later, Knox and Carrigan reported that four of six adult patients with AIDS had areas of demyelination (loss of the insulating sheaths of nerve cells that make up white matter) in their brain tissues at the time of their deaths, and HHV-6 infected cells were found only in areas of demyelination.[26]

Still more convincingly, ten of ten lymph node biopsy samples taken from early asymptomatic HIV-positive people were found infected with HHV-6, even though their CD4 T-cell counts were above the clinical AIDS level (one had 711 CD4 T-cells/μl).[27] That meant HHV-6 was clearly active before AIDS had even been diagnosed. In contrast, no lymph node biopsy sample from HIV-negative controls was infected with HHV-6.

Knox and Carrigan also found HHV-6 infections in people who died of AIDS-like symptoms who were HIV-negative, as described in detail by Nicholas Regush, a journalist who championed their work in his book *The Virus Within*.[28]

HIV DOES NOT CAUSE AIDS

The findings described in this and earlier chapters vindicate what AIDS dissidents such as Peter Duesberg and David Rasnick have been saying all along: HIV does not necessarily cause AIDS. AIDS disease can occur in the absence of HIV; conversely, HIV-positive people need not develop AIDS disease. Furthermore, AIDS may be a "genomics disease" resulting from drug use or exposure to toxic agents in the environment that scramble the genome and wake up lethal viruses.

Predictably, the AIDS research establishment has remained hostile to such ideas, and there is little or no funding for Knox and Carrigan's work, nor, until very recently, that of Urnovitz or any other approach to prevention or therapy.

Away from the glare of acrimonious debates, other scientists have quietly adopted a different approach to vaccine development and are claiming striking success, as we shall see in the next chapter.

The "Pink Panacea":
An AIDS Vaccine?

AN UNCONVENTIONAL VACCINE COULD PROVIDE TREATMENT FOR AIDS.

AN ORAL VACCINE THAT TARGETS MUCOSAL IMMUNITY

A company based in Thailand has developed an oral vaccine against HIV/AIDS. The makers of a pink pill called "V1" claim striking success in the treatment of HIV/AIDS symptoms.[1]

Immunitor Corporation Company and V1's creators are clinical researcher Dr. Aldar S. Bourinbaiar and pharmacist Vichai Jirathitikal, who have put V1 through a placebo-controlled phase II study. The results showed significant improvements in CD4 and CD8 cell counts, weight gain, decreased viral load, and survival of end-stage AIDS patients. The trial also suggested that V1 could reverse the progression of AIDS without concurrent toxicity.[2]

Immunitor and Dr. Orapun Metadilogkul, an independent physician who heads the Thailand Association of Occupational and Environmental Medicine Physicians, claim that twenty-seven patients diagnosed with HIV/AIDS have changed from HIV-positive to HIV-negative after treatment with V1. A phase III trial application has been submitted to the Thai Food and Drug Administration aimed at demonstrating the beneficial properties of V1 on associated symptoms of AIDS such as wasting. If approved, trials will take place at the largest public hospital in Bangkok under Dr. Metadilogkul.

V1 is said to be a therapeutic vaccine comprising "HIV antigens from pooled clinical isolates from HIV-infected donors." These antigens are made into pills taken orally that do not degrade in the digestion process of the stomach but trigger immune responses in the underlying mucosa-associated immune cells in the lining of the small intestine.

Some 90 percent of the immune cells in the human body are made up of lymphocytes and monocytes in the lining of the mucosal surfaces. This means there are ten times more CD4 and CD8 lymphocytes—crucial in the immune response against AIDS—residing in the mucosal lining than in the blood, where only 2 percent of lymphocytes are present. According to Immunitor, these intestinal cells are the front-line defense against HIV and are the first to be destroyed or disabled by the virus.

Once mucosal immunity has failed, the common and often fatal symptoms of HIV/AIDS appear, such as diarrhea and respiratory infections. V1 works on the premise that HIV/AIDS is a disease of mucosal immunity, so targeting antigens at mucosal surfaces is a valid clinical approach (see "Vaccinating People Against Their Own Genes").

FREE VACCINATIONS AT MASS RALLIES

Public opinion on V1 came sharply into focus when Thai clinics began giving out the pink pills free of charge to AIDS patients at mass rallies organized in schools, police stations, sport stadiums, and Buddhist temples. There was opposition to these actions by those working in conventional medical practices, despite the fact that they have no effective treatment to offer to patients with HIV/AIDS.

V1 has been extensively subjected to toxicity studies both *in vitro* and *in vivo*. So far, studies by the Thai government and independent private laboratories have proved it exhibits no toxicity. Five mammalian cell lines tested at the highest dose of 10mg/ml showed no sign of cytotoxicity. The extrapolated dose of V1 that would cause death in humans is 2,200 pills per day, as against the recommended daily dose for adults of one pill per day.

FIRST RESULTS ENCOURAGING

Recently published data from Immunitor show that forty AIDS patients on a six-month trial of V1 treatment increased their CD4 and CD8 cell counts by a mean average of fifty-one cells (19 percent) per microliter of blood. Increase in body weight was 2.2 kg on average. But some patients' weight increased by as much as 30 kg, which is an important gain in the treatment of AIDS.

These encouraging results led Bourinbaiar and Jirathitikal to evaluate V1 therapy in the treatment of terminally ill AIDS patients in intensive care wards in Thai hospitals. They approached 117 patients; 53 decided to take V1, while 64 declined treatment. All patients were bedridden and had been receiving palliative care. None of the patients had access to conventional antiretroviral drugs, but some had been treated with antibiotics. All the patients in the non-V1 group were dead by week nine. In contrast, 30 of the 53 in the V1 group were alive and able to resume normal activity.

After twenty months on V1, 18 percent of the remaining patients, who had started with almost zero CD4 counts, were still alive. It was also noted that patients receiving V1 seldom developed opportunistic infections, which further suggests that V1 improves mucosal immune responses to infections.

A retrospective analysis by Bourinbaiar and Jirathitikal of 650 HIV-positive patients who had taken V1 for an average of twenty-three weeks showed significant results. In total, 496 patients (76 percent) were able to increase their body weight, or at least maintain weight, on the V1 regime; 389 (59 percent) gained 4.2 kg, while 107 (17 percent) remained unchanged and 159 (24 percent) lost weight. Everyone participating in the trial was able to remain on it and suffered no serious side effects.[3]

A further study took place in which V1 was administered to the HIV-negative relatives of terminally ill AIDS patients over a median period of twenty-four days. Their blood was then transfused into the AIDS patients, who experienced an improvement in their health. Results showed that increases in CD4 and CD8 counts were statistically significant.[4]

LICENSED AS FOOD SUPPLEMENT

V1 is currently licensed as a food supplement by the Thai Food and Drug Administration and is produced for research and development purposes. A one-month supply costs around £20 to £30 ($38 to $57) per person, but it is given freely to poor patients in public hospitals wherever possible. So far, 65,000 Thais infected with HIV have been given the treatment.

Costs for V1 contrast strikingly with those of more established combination therapies or "cocktails" consisting of three-drug antiretrovirals for the treatment of HIV/AIDS. A recent HIV Cost Services Utilization Study Consortium Analysis estimates that in the United States, 33,500 HIV-infected adults seen twice a year for medications and blood tests spend $6.7 billion, or $22,000 per patient, per year.[5]

Apart from the economic viability of V1, there may be other advantages when considering its use as a safe therapy for the developing world. It has broad-spectrum activity against many HIV subtypes and is stable in ambient tropical temperatures for three years, making refrigeration unnecessary. And because it is in pill form, no special skills or equipment is needed to administer it.[6]

Immunitor has not disclosed the medicinal properties of VI, but instead recommends a cocktail of V1 and certain generic drugs as alternative and inexpensive treatments for HIV/AIDS. Immunitor cites examples of five compounds: gramicidin (the first antibiotic to be isolated), cimetidine (Tagamet), warfarin (a common anticoagulant), levamisole (an animal dewormer, originally developed for animal use, but recently become a useful drug in treating colon cancer in humans), and acetaminophen (paracetamol). Immunitor says these unapproved drugs are all highly effective against HIV/AIDS,[7] and they are extremely inexpensive in comparison to approved combination therapies.

Clinical trials of V1 are ongoing, and phase III trials are scheduled for Africa with results pending. V1 is registered in Ghana, and licenses have been applied for in several other African states. Immunitor hopes to build a vaccine plant to supply large amounts of V1 to Africans at low cost. This would meet a critical demand for affordable and available HIV/AIDS treatment on the African continent.

POVERTY AND AIDS TREATMENT

Much attention is centered on the apparently high rates of infection and death, 95 percent, attributed to HIV/AIDS in the developing world. But until recently the intimate association between the pandemic and poverty has been played down in the application of strategic approaches for

HIV/AIDS. In a recent letter to *The Times* of London, Prof. Kenneth Stuart, the medical advisor to the Commonwealth Secretariat, highlighted the need to recognize the role of poverty in effective treatments for HIV/AIDS. He wrote, "The more the gap widens between rich and poor the greater the number of people who are left stranded in the backwaters of progress." So not only are people in poverty traps deprived access to helpful technologies and medicines, their ability to acquire knowledge is diminished, along with their human rights.[8]

The report "Thailand Social Monitor: Poverty and Public Policy" says 16 percent of the country's population, or about 10 million people, are now living on less than the minimal income of Bt900 ($21.78) per person per month, which constitutes the country's poverty line.[9]

"Poverty is re-emerging as one of the nation's most serious problems," said Ian Porter, the World Bank's country director for Thailand, at the launch of the new report, which was jointly prepared by the National Economic and Social Development Board, the Thailand Development Research Institute, and international experts.[10] An international AIDS conference was held in Bangkok in July 2004.

In the next chapter we shall see how malnutrition and undernutrition associated with poverty compromise the immune system, leaving populations vulnerable to infection and disease.

Eating Well for Health

EATING WELL IS NECESSARY FOR MAINTAINING A BALANCED
IMMUNE SYSTEM THAT PROTECTS US FROM DISEASE AND
RESTORES THE BODY TO HEALTH.

NUTRITION AND IMMUNITY

A balanced immune system is vital for keeping the body healthy, and good nutrition is the key. This is the overwhelming message of scientific research over the past decade, brought home in numerous reviews.[1-4]

Undernutrition impairs the immune system, suppressing immune functions that are fundamental to host defense. Undernutrition can be due to insufficient food—energy and macronutrients, such as carbohydrates, protein, and nucleic acids—or due to deficiencies in specific micronutrients, vitamins, co-factors, and minerals. Macro- and micronutrient deficiencies often occur together, particularly in poor third world countries (see box).

Apparently well-fed and overfed populations in industrialized countries may nevertheless suffer from micronutrient deficiencies due to soil depletion from years of intensive industrial monoculture food-farming.

A comparison of mineral content in British food produce—carrots, potatoes, cauliflower, celery, chicken, beef, lamb, pork, and cod—between 1936 (before the introduction of industrial agriculture) and 1987 showed that there were overall 49 percent more minerals in food produced in 1936.[5] The most-depleted minerals were iron, magnesium, and calcium. Calcium and iron deficiencies are prevalent among young people today. Iron and magnesium are both important for the maintenance of immunity (see below).

> ## World Malnutrition and Undernutrition
>
> - Almost 800 million people (one-sixth of the population of the world's developing nations) are malnourished, 200 million of them children.
> - In developing nations, one in four persons lacks access to safe drinking water.
> - Seven hundred and ninety million people in the developing world, and 34 million people in the industrialized world, mostly in the former Soviet Union, are chronically undernourished.
> - There are 185.9 million hungry people in sub-Saharan Africa, or 34 percent of the population.
>
> **Source:** Food and Agriculture Organization

Nutrients that have been demonstrated (in animal or human studies) to be required for immune function include the essential amino acids, the essential fatty acids linoleic acid and alpha-linolenic acid, vitamin A, folic acid, vitamin B_6, vitamin B_{12}, vitamin C, vitamin E, zinc, copper, iron, and selenium. Practically all forms of immunity may be affected by deficiencies in one or more of these nutrients. Animal and human studies have demonstrated that adding the deficient nutrient back to the diet can restore immune function and resistance to infection.

In protein–energy malnutrition, experienced by starving populations in many third world countries and especially in sub-Saharan Africa, bacterial and/or viral infections represent the major cause of death. Protein–energy malnutrition impairs immune defense against infectious diseases through undermining skin and mucosal barriers, depletion of lymphocytes, reduction of phagocytic functions, and defects in T-cells due to the failure of macrophages to produce interleukin-1. Furthermore, the thymus atrophies—probably through stress-induced steroid production—contributing to the general impairment of cell-mediated immunity.

Micronutrient deficiencies and infectious disease often coexist and show complex interactions leading to mutually reinforced detrimental clinical effects. Micronutrient deficiency, in general, has a widespread effect on nearly all components of the innate immune response.

VITAMINS

Vitamin A deficiency is a major public health problem in many developing countries: up to 10 million children shows signs of deficiency, and an estimated 100 million children are subclinically depleted. Vitamin A deficiency is associated with increased frequency of infections, especially through a severe impairment of antibody-mediated immunity, or Th2 humoral immune response (see "Vaccinating People Against Their Own Genes"). Providing vitamin A supplements has been found to improve the antibody response to measles vaccine, maintain gut integrity, lower the incidence of respiratory tract infections, and reduce mortality associated with diarrhea and measles.[6] There are clinical data suggesting that vitamin A deficiency in HIV-1–infected individuals contributes to mortality, disease progression, and maternal–infant disease transfer (see "The 'Pink Panacea': An AIDS Vaccine?"). WHO has recommended that vitamin A supplements should be given to all individuals in developing countries who contract measles. In animal models, vitamin A deficiency produced a host of immune dysfunctions, including the inhibition of mitogen-stimulated T-cell proliferation, antigen-specific antibody production, and the ability to produce immunoglobulin (Ig) A and Ig G. It also reduced the ability of CD4 cells to provide the B-cell stimulus for antigen-specific IgG responses. Most of the effects were reversed with restoration of vitamin A.

Vitamin C is an antioxidant that is highly concentrated in white blood cells to reduce auto-oxidation of phagocytes and damage to other cells without compromising the oxidative capacity of phagocytes. Deficiency in vitamin C is associated with decreased resistance to infection and cancer, reduced phagocytosis, and impairment of T-cell–mediated immune responses and wound repair. There has been a longstanding debate concerning the possibility that high doses of vitamin C can boost immunity. According to some researchers, "a wealth of epidemiological studies suggest that higher intakes of vitamin C and other antioxidants are associated with a lower risk of chronic diseases such as cancer and cardiovascular disease,"[7] but few of these studies measured specific immune components. Vitamin C has been shown to have some clinical effects in the treatment of autoimmune diseases, allergy, asthma, and immune-suppressive disorders, including HIV.

Vitamin E and selenium act synergistically in tissues to reduce damage to lipid membranes by reactive oxygen species formed during infections. Vitamin E deficiency is considered quite rare in human beings; under experimental conditions, deficiency of vitamin E causes reduced functions of T-cells and phagocytes, and decreased tumor resistance. Vitamin E supplements increased Th1 functions and reduced oxidative damage.[8]

Vitamin D stimulates the development of monocytes and macrophages as well as their phagocytosis.

MINERALS

Zinc deficiency is very common among populations whose diet is based on cereals, which contain low levels of zinc. Deficiency of zinc is known to occur in many disease states, including alcoholism, renal disease, burns, and gastrointestinal tract disorders, as well as HIV-AIDS and diarrhea. Zinc deficiency reduces the thymus and causes abnormalities in T-cells. In particular, Th1, Th2, and cytotoxic T-lymphocyte functions are all depressed. Zinc is required for the oxidative burst of macrophages during destruction of pathogens. It is also required in transcription factors and hormone receptors in the nucleus. It is required for the activity of more than 100 enzymes in core metabolism. Balb/C mice (a laboratory strain) fed a zinc-deficient diet for eight days suffered 80 percent mortality when infected with a sublethal dose of *Trypanosoma cruzi* (causing Chagas disease), compared with 10 percent mortality in control mice.[9]

Selenium is an essential component of glutathione peroxidase (GP), and in collaboration with vitamin E, it prevents the peroxidation of cell and membrane lipids. In particular, GP produced by phagocytes prevents auto-oxidation and tissue damage due to excess hydrogen peroxide generated. Selenium may also be involved in post-translational modifications of proteins related to the immune system, such as CD4 and CD8. Selenium deficiency impairs antibody and cytokine production, lymphocyte proliferation, and the cell-killing capacity of cytotoxic

T-lymphocytes. Mice with severe selenium deficiency since birth and control mice were infected with a sublethal dose of *Trypanosoma cruzi*. Only the selenium-deficient mice died during the acute-phase inflammatory response with multiple organ failure, while the control, selenium-sufficient mice survived, indicating that selenium plays an important role in regulating the inflammatory response.[10]

Copper deficiency is associated with increased susceptibility to infection in animals and humans, probably due to a severe depression of phagocytic and T-cell functions, especially the reduced production of interleukin-2. Copper is implicated in complement function, cell membrane integrity, copper-selenium superoxide dismutase and immunoglobulin structure.

Iron deficit is estimated to affect 20 to 50 percent of the world's population, making it the most widespread nutritional deficiency.[11] Iron deficiency is characterized by impaired proliferation of Th1 cells, and hence cell-mediated immune functions. Iron is required by hemoglobin, the oxygen carrier of red blood cells, and many key metalloenzymes in energy metabolism. Many of the immune abnormalities associated with iron deficiency appear to be reversible with iron supplement. Although iron is essential for the immune system, too much is toxic. Iron overload impairs many immune functions, including causing a decrease in antibody-mediated and mitogen-stimulated phagocytosis by monocytes and macrophages, a reduction of neutrophil migration, disturbances of T-lymphocyte distribution and function, and an increased rate of infections.

During the past few years, magnesium has emerged as one of the most important micronutrients to the immune system, strongly affecting both innate and adaptive immunity.[12]

LIPIDS

Dietary fatty acids affect vital cellular functions such as energy metabolism, signaling, oxidation, and membrane fluidity. Arachidonic acid is a fundamental constituent of membrane phospholipids; its metabolism gives rise to molecules that act as immunosuppressants that down-regulate Th1 cells and promote immunoglobulin synthesis. In general, a high content of fatty acids in the diet causes immunosuppression, and saturated fats are thought to play a major role in inhibiting the immune system. (But see articles on the Web site of the Weston A. Price Foundation for an alternative view that is gaining ground, www.westonaprice.org/knowyourfats/fats_lungs.html.)

Long-chain polyunsaturated fatty acids (PUFAs) include the essential fatty acids, linoleic and alpha-linolenic acids (chain of eighteen carbons, with two and three double-bonds respectively), which cannot be synthesized by mammalian cells and must be obtained from the diet. Linoleic acid is found in most plant oils and animal fats, whereas alpha-linolenic acid is found in flax seed, soybean, and canola oils. Longer-chain PUFAs such as arachidonic acid (twenty carbons, four double bonds), eicosapentaeonic acid (EPA, twenty carbons, five double bonds), and docosahexaenoic acid (DHA, twenty-two carbons, six double bonds) can be synthesized from alpha-linolenic acid in humans and can also be obtained from marine fish oils. These lipids are important in brain development, cardiovascular disease, and cancer; and there is now evidence that dietary PUFA, particularly EPA and DHA, have a major impact on many immune functions.[13]

Fish-oil supplement in clinical trials and animal models of rheumatoid arthritis, ulcerative colitis, psoriasis, and organ transplant has resulted in measurable benefits on the immune system. Feeding fish oil to animals reduces disease severity and prolongs survival in animal models of lupus. Fish-oil supplement suppresses inflammatory/autoimmune responses, and excessive levels given to healthy subjects may reduce survival or pathogen clearance.

PROTEINS AND NUCLEIC ACID

Protein deprivation leads to a severe depression of the immune response. Many body functions, such as tissue homeostasis and repair, cell proliferation, and production of inflammatory mediators are impaired in protein deprivation.

Nucleotides are obtained from nucleoprotein-rich foods such as organ meats, fish, and poultry and are especially high in human breast milk. Nucleotides are the building blocks for DNA and RNA and are involved in major energy transduction and signaling processes. Nucleotide-free diets affect many immune responses, including decreased natural killer cell and macrophage activity, decreased interleukin-2 production, interferon-γ release and phagocytic functions, and increased susceptibility to infections. Addition of nucleotides to nucleotide-free diets has been shown to reverse many of the changes associated with nucleotide deficiency.

MICRONUTRIENT DEFICIENCIES AND VIRULENCE OF PATHOGENS

The association between viral disease and nutrition has long been attributed solely to effects on the host immune system. A remarkable study showed, however, that the virus itself could also be affected by the nutritional status of the host. Researchers at the University of North Carolina demonstrated that a normally benign strain of coxsackievirus B3 (CVB3/0) became virulent in either selenium-deficient or vitamin E–deficient mice.[14] Although the nutritionally deficient animals were immunosuppressed, the virus itself became altered. Six nucleotide changes were found in the virus that replicated in the deficient mice, and once these mutations occurred, even mice with normal nutritional status became susceptible to disease when tested. As both selenium and vitamin E act as antioxidants, it is thought that oxidative stress in the deficient mice may have caused the genetic changes in the virus. The benign virus injected into GP–knockout mice (which can no longer get rid of free radicals effectively) also converted to virulence due to genomic changes. It appears that the GP enzyme is essential for preventing damage to the RNA-viral genome that results in the mutations.

This finding has significant implications for epidemiology. Poor nutritional status in individuals may start epidemics among the entire population, even though the rest of the population is not nutritionally deficient.

AGING, IMMUNITY, AND NUTRITION

Aging is characterized by a decline in a broad spectrum of immune functions, a process referred to as immunosenescence, which may account for the increased frequency of infections, cancers, and autoimmune diseases among older people.

Immunosenescence includes the inability of aged CD8 cells, natural killer cells, and B-cells to be activated by superantigens. These and other changes are similar to findings in HIV-infected patients (see "Vaccinating People Against Their Own Genes"). These parallels led to the suggestion that "HIV-infection, via a process of chronic immune activation, might accelerate the ageing of the immune system."[15]

In other words, AIDS may be a disease of an overstressed, exhausted immune system.

Other researchers point out that the changes in aging are mainly related to health status and are more important in the undernourished elderly, in the elderly deficient in micronutrients, and even more so in elderly patients with protein–energy malnutrition. Seniors with protein–energy malnutrition showed decreased immune functions for all aspects of immunity: T-cell and B-cell subsets and functions and innate immunity.[16]

In a study comparing adaptive and innate immunity in healthy and generally well-nourished elderly women (sixty-two to eighty-eight years old) with younger women (twenty to forty years old), no differences in total T-cell, T-helper (CD4) cell, or T-cytotoxic (CD8) cell numbers were detected, although older women tended to have lower T-cell proliferation response to stimulation with the mitogens (substances that stimulate cell division) concanavalin A and especially phytohemagglutinin.[17] There were no age-related changes in natural killer cell number or cytotoxicity; and phagocytosis and subsequent oxidative burst activity also did not differ between the younger and older women. Most immune parameters showed no decline with aging in this group of apparently healthy, well-nourished women.

This study suggests that nutritional intervention can reduce immune dysfunction among the elderly and hence their risk of infection. Indeed, nutritional therapy is now a well-established intervention in many diseases, including AIDS (see the next chapter).

PROBIOTICS

No discussion on nutrition today is complete without mentioning probiotics. These are bacteria that have beneficial effects on the health and well-being of the host.[18] They are not nutrients strictly speaking but are increasingly recognized to be important to immunity. A great diversity of such bacteria live in the human gut and other mucosal surfaces, less than half of which can be cultured and identified. The main action of probiotics is to reinforce the mucosal barrier against harmful agents. This includes reducing pathological changes that increase the permeability of the gut to large molecules or bacteria, stimulating mucosal immunity, reducing mucus degradation, and preventing inflammation.[19]

Mucosal immune response begins at birth, and responses generated at this time support specific immunity in later life. Lactating mammary glands are part of an integrated mucosal immune system in which antibodies—mainly IgA—are produced locally. These antibodies reflect antigenic stimulation of mucosa-associated lymphoid tissues by common intestinal and respiratory pathogens. Antibodies in breast milk are thus highly targeted against infectious agents in the mother's environment, and breast-feeding serves a vital function in protecting the child against infections. Mucosal pathogens are a major killer of children below the age of five years; they are responsible for more than 14 million deaths annually. Diarrheal disease alone takes a toll of 5 million children a year in developing countries. Epidemiological data suggest that the risk of dying from diarrhea could be reduced fourteen to twenty-four times if all children were breast-fed.[20]

Because mucosal immunity is modulated by the interaction of the gut microflora (bacteria and yeasts) with the gut immune system, probiotics can play a major role in stimulating the mucosal immune system. A study was conducted in a periurban population in south Delhi in India on 634 children randomly allocated to either receiving milk formula containing the probiotic bacterium *Bifidobacterium lactis* HN019 plus galacto-oligosaccharides, or the same milk without the two added.[21] The results showed that children receiving the probiotic supplement in milk had a significant reduction in dysentery, days of severe illness, fever, and ear infections. Iron deficiency was reduced by 35 percent, and the children showed significantly better growth at six months and one year.

In a randomized double-blind, placebo-controlled clinical trial involving twenty-five elderly volunteers taking 180ml low-fat/low-lactose milk twice daily for a period of six weeks, the thirteen test subjects who had milk supplemented with *Bifidobacterium lactis* were found to have enhanced natural immunity.[22] They had significant increase in polymorphonuclear cell phagocytic capacity and enhanced phagocyte-mediated bactericidal activity. The peripheral blood mononuclear cells from test subjects also produced enhanced levels of interferon-α (an antiviral cytokine) upon stimulation.

Despite this wealth of evidence linking nutritional status and immunity, there have been relatively few studies on nutritional therapy against HIV/AIDS.

New results from a study showing that multivitamin supplementation can delay disease progression and death in HIV-positive women in Tanzania raises serious questions over the ethics of the current global initiative to fight HIV/AIDS that focuses on anti-HIV drugs and vaccines, as we shall see in the next chapter.

Eating Well
Against HIV/AIDS

RESULTS OF THE FIRST CLINICAL TRIALS SUGGEST THAT NUTRITIONAL SUPPLEMENTS CAN DELAY DISEASE PROGRESSION AND DEATH IN HIV-POSITIVE PEOPLE, ESPECIALLY IN THIRD WORLD COUNTRIES.

MULTIVITAMINS AGAINST HIV

A trial of multivitamin supplements on HIV disease progression and mortality was published in the *New England Journal of Medicine* in July 2004.[1] It involved 1,078 pregnant women infected with HIV enrolled in Dar es Salaam, Tanzania, followed up for a median of seventy-one months (range forty-six to eighty months). The results show that improving the nutritional status of HIV-positive women can delay disease progression and death.

Of 271 women who received multivitamins, 67 (24.7 percent) progressed to stage 4 disease or died, compared with 83 of 267 women (31.1 percent) who received placebo. Multivitamin supplementation reduced the relative risk of death and of progression to stage 4 disease, or progression to stage 3 or higher. It also resulted in significantly higher CD4 and CD8 cell counts and significantly lower viral loads.

Multivitamin supplementation had many other benefits. It significantly reduced oral and gastrointestinal manifestations of HIV disease and reduced reported fatigue, rash, and acute upper respiratory tract infections. Multivitamins also significantly reduced all signs of complications, including oral ulcers, angular cheilitis (painful cracking and soreness that develops at the corners of the mouth), difficult or painful swallowing, dysentery, and fatigue.

The trial included vitamin A intake, but the results showed that the effects of vitamin A alone were smaller and for the most part not significantly different from those produced by placebo as far as disease progression and death were concerned. Adding vitamin A to the multivitamin regimen *reduced* the benefit with regard to some of the end points examined. Vitamin A supplement, as compared with no vitamin A supplement, also increased the relative risks of angular cheilitis and difficult or painful swallowing and resulted in significantly lower CD8 cell counts.

The study, carried out jointly by Harvard Medical School in Boston and Muhimbili University College of Health Sciences in Dar es Salaam, Tanzania, has been ongoing since 1995. It is the clearest result, so far, that multivitamin supplement can delay the progression to AIDS disease. The researchers, quite rationally, recommend it as "an effective, low-cost means of delaying the initiation of antiretroviral therapy in HIV-infected women."

The researchers point out that the timing of the initiation of antiretroviral therapy is still controversial (due to the many side effects; see the chapter "Anti-HIV Drugs Do More Harm Than Good"). The revised U.S. guidelines for adults recommend starting when AIDS-related symptoms develop or, for asymptomatic adults, when CD4 cell counts drop below 350 per cubic millimeter, or plasma levels of HIV-type RNA exceed 55,000 copies per milliliter.[2] Introducing multivitamin supplements would save antiretroviral drugs for later use, avoid adverse events associated with them, and significantly reduce treatment-related costs as well. A year's supply of the multivitamins used in this trial is approximately $15 per person, and the wholesale price is substantially lower.

A somewhat skeptical editorial in the same issue of the *New England Journal of Medicine* accompanied its publication of the study, pointing out that there was a need to confirm the new findings and to evaluate the effects of multivitamins in larger populations.[3]

Nevertheless, the editorial admits, "As donor-funded initiatives expand in Africa, it has become clear that nutrition will have to be addressed in the treatment of HIV disease and AIDS."

The editorial's authors confess that in the focus-group discussions they conducted when starting an antiretroviral treatment program in a large Nairobi slum, every group interviewed said the lack of food was the most likely cause of nonadherence to antiretroviral (ARV) drug therapy, probably because it made the side effects of the drugs more difficult to endure. One participant in a focus group was reported to have said, "If you give us ARVs, please give us food, just food."

Indeed, the study raises many other questions. Would the results have been even better if the women were given food *in addition* to multivitamin supplements? Could the women be suffering from protein–energy malnutrition and other micronutrient deficits? Could that be why they failed to benefit from vitamin A? Why has it taken so long for vitamin supplements to be given? And why is food supplement *still* not given to the women in this study, or indeed routinely given with ARVs?

This study came in the wake of accumulating evidence that micronutrient deficits are associated with AIDS disease progression and HIV infection, and some indications that micronutrient supplements, including vitamins and minerals, may slow the development of AIDS disease.

HIV AND NUTRITION

There is already a wealth of evidence (reviewed in the previous chapter) that adequate nutrition is necessary for the development and maintenance of immunity against infections and disease. Nutritional status and immunity are intimately connected (see previous chapter), and a wide range of nutritional deficiencies, from protein–energy malnutrition to deficits of micronutrients, can leave the body susceptible to infections. A similar picture has emerged in HIV/AIDS.

Analysis of vitamin A levels, CD4 T-cells, complete blood cell count, and serologic markers for liver disease was carried out in a random subsample of 179 subjects from a cohort of more than 2,000 recreational intravenous drug users in the United States, with longitudinal follow-up to determine survival. The follow-up time was 22.8 ± 1.1 months, during which 15 subjects died. More than 15 percent of the HIV-positive individuals had plasma vitamin A levels less than 1.05 micromol/L (vitamin A deficient). The HIV-positive individuals had lower mean plasma vitamin A levels than HIV-negative individuals. Vitamin A deficiency was associated with lower CD4 counts among both seronegative and seropositive individuals. In the HIV-seropositive participants, vitamin A deficiency was associated with increased mortality (relative risk = 6.3; 95 percent confidence interval, 2.1 to 18.6).[4]

Serum from forty-seven HIV-seropositive patients was evaluated for micronutrients. Comparisons were made between groups divided by different CD4 cell count and whether the subjects were suffering from wasting syndrome. The results showed that mean serum levels were significantly lower for vitamin A, folate, and carotene in patients with wasting syndrome than in nonwasting syndrome patients with comparable CD4 cell counts. Values of vitamins A, B_6, C, D, carotene and reduced glutathione (GSH, the body's own antioxidant) were below normal in over 10 percent of HIV-seropositive patients. The researchers noted that particular deficiencies might be only part of the larger picture of malabsorption and undernutrition.[5]

In a survey carried out on vitamin supplement use and nutritional status in sixty-four HIV-seropositive men and women and thirty-three seronegative controls in the United States, HIV-infected subjects were found to have significantly lower mean circulating concentrations of magnesium, carotenes, choline, and GSH, but significantly higher concentrations of niacin (water-soluble components of the vitamin B complex) than controls. Fifty-nine percent of HIV-positive subjects had low concentrations of magnesium, compared with 9 percent of controls. These abnormal concentrations were unrelated to stage of AIDS disease. Participants who took vitamin supplements had consistently fewer low concentrations of antioxidants, irrespective of HIV infection status and disease stage.[6]

Twenty-nine percent of the HIV-positive subjects taking vitamin supplements nevertheless had subnormal levels of one or more antioxidants. The researchers suggested that frequent occurrence of abnormal micronutrient levels, as found in these HIV-positive subjects, might contribute to AIDS disease, and that the low magnesium concentrations might be particularly relevant to HIV-related symptoms of fatigue, lethargy, and impaired thinking.

Another study in the United States involved one hundred and six HIV-infected outpatients and twenty-nine uninfected control subjects (eighty-nine men and forty-six women; age range: thirty-five to fifty-seven years). The HIV-infected subjects represented a broad range of disease progression. Lower concentrations of plasma and erythrocyte (red blood cell) magnesium and of erythrocyte GSH were found in HIV-infected subjects, beginning early in the course of HIV-1 infection. There were significant associations between the CD4 T-lymphocyte count and hematocrit (number and size of red blood cells), plasma magnesium concentration, and plasma zinc concentration. The lowest erythrocyte magnesium concentrations occurred in HIV-infected subjects who consumed alcoholic beverages. Independent variables that were significant joint predictors of CD4 cell count were hematocrit and plasma choline and zinc concentrations. The results, again, provided evidence that compromised nutritional and antioxidant status begin early in the course of HIV-1 infection and may contribute to disease progression.[7]

A fifth study followed 108 HIV-1-seropositive homosexual men for eighteen months following their initial diagnosis. The results showed that the development of deficiency of vitamin A or vitamin B_{12} was associated with a decline in CD4 cell count, while normalization of vitamin A, vitamin B_{12}, and zinc was associated with higher CD4 cell counts, irrespective of AZT use. For vitamin B_{12}, low baseline status significantly predicted accelerated HIV-1 disease progression.[8]

Taken altogether, the findings suggest that micronutrient deficiencies are associated with HIV-1 disease progression and possibly also with infection.

The findings in HIV-positive children were similar. A study in France revealed significant deficiencies of lycopene and retinal (vitamin A precursors), tocopherol (vitamin E), transthyretin (a serum protein that transports thyroxine and retinol-binding protein), and serum albumin in twenty-one HIV-positive children, compared to twenty-one matched controls (ages two to nine years). The HIV-positive children were divided into two groups according to whether they had developed AIDS disease. The deficiencies were there before disease developed and persisted in the disease state.[9] Neither transthyretin nor serum albumin is a micronutrient, but they are indicators of health. Albumin is the protein present in the highest concentration in plasma, and it transports many small molecules in the blood (for example, calcium, progesterone, and drugs) and prevents fluid from leaking out from the bloodstream into the tissues. A low concentration of serum albumin is a sign of liver or kidney disease.[10]

A subsequent report from Italy on twenty children one to six years old with HIV infection found "a state of hypovitaminosis [vitamin deficiency] involving the most important antioxidant vitamins."[11]

A research team followed 474 HIV-infected mothers and their infants in Malawi, from pregnancy through to the infants' twelfth month of life.

Of the 474 HIV-infected pregnant women, 300 (63.3 percent) were deficient in vitamin A (serum level less than 1.05 micromol/L). The mean serum vitamin A levels among mothers whose infants died were 0.78 ± 0.03 micromol/L, compared with 1.02 ± 0.02 micromol/L among mothers whose infants had survived for the first twelve months. The overall infant mortality rate was 28.7 percent. The HIV-positive mothers were divided into six groups according to serum vitamin A levels, from the lowest to the highest: group 1, less than 0.35; group 2, between 0.35 and 0.70; group 3, between 0.70 and 1.05; group 4, between 1.05 and 1.40; group 5, between 1.40 and 1.75; and group 6, more than 1.75. Infant mortality rates for each group were 93.3 percent, 41.6 percent, 23.4 percent, 18.5 percent, 17.7 percent, and 14.2 percent, respectively.[12] This strongly suggested that maternal vitamin A deficiency during HIV infection could contribute to increased infant mortality.

NOURISHING AGAINST AIDS

The idea of nutritional therapy for AIDS arose in the holistic health community on the grounds that malnutrition can exacerbate immunosuppression, and that therefore, by maintaining the HIV-infected with optimum nutrition, AIDS disease can be delayed or ameliorated.[13] The recommendation to take a one-a-day vitamin supplement is the simplest form of nutritional therapy, while tube feeding and drip-feed might be required in the seriously ill. However, large doses or "megadoses" of vitamins and minerals were to be avoided, as they could impair immunity and be otherwise harmful.

Nutritional therapy was also recommended as an adjunct to AIDS treatment to overcome the toxic effects of conventional anti-HIV drugs.[14] For example, L-carnitine and acetyl-L-carnitine have been used in treating mitochondrial toxicity, both in muscle and nerve pathologies, because the anti-HIV nucleoside analog reverse transcriptase (RT) inhibitor is toxic to mitochondria.

MICRONUTRIENTS *IN VITRO*

Some micronutrients appear to have effects on viral RT, as indicated by the results of experiments carried out *in vitro* (in the test tube).

Ascorbic acid (vitamin C) and its calcium salt (Ca-ascorbate), and two antioxidants, GSH and N-acetyl-L-cysteine (NAC), were tested in chronically HIV-1 infected T-lymphocytes.[15] Ca-ascorbate reduced extracellular HIV RT activity by about the same magnitude as the equivalent dose of ascorbic acid. Continuous presence of ascorbate was necessary for suppressing HIV. NAC caused a less than twofold inhibition of HIV RT and conferred a synergistic effect (approximately eightfold inhibition) when tested simultaneously with ascorbic acid. In contrast, GSH had no effect on RT concentrations and did not potentiate the anti-HIV effect of ascorbate. A concentration of 300 micrograms/ml ascorbate resulted in approximately five- to ten-fold inhibition of extracellular RT activity stimulated by the cytokine TNF-γ.[16] These results support the potent antiviral activity of ascorbate and suggest its therapeutic value in controlling HIV infection in combination with antioxidants.

In another experiment, forty-four different metal ions were tested for their *in vitro* effects on the activity of the RT of HIV-1.[17] Five of the metal ions—Pt^{4+} (platinum), Ag^+ (silver), Rh^{3+} (rhodium), Zn^{2+} (zinc), and Hg^{2+} (mercury)—were found to inhibit the RT activity in a dose-dependent manner. The order of effectiveness was $Pt^{4+} > Ag^+ > Rh^{3+} > Zn^{2+} = Hg^{2+}$. Estimated mean concentrations for 50 percent inhibition (IC50) were 7.8 microM for platinum, 14.1 microM for silver, 46.8 microM for rhodium, 53.7 microM for zinc, and 56.2 microM for mercury.

VITAMIN SUPPLEMENTS *IN VIVO*

The trial on pregnant HIV-positive women carried out in Tanzania, described at the beginning of this chapter, started in 1995. The birth outcomes of the women were reported in 1998.[18] There were thirty fetal deaths (11.15 percent) among 269 women taking multivitamins compared with forty-nine (18.35 percent) among the 267 women not on multivitamins. Multivitamin supplement decreased the risk of low birth weight (less than 2,500 g) by 44 percent, severe preterm birth (less than 34 weeks' gestation) by 39 percent, and small size for gestational age at birth by 43 percent. Vitamin A supplement, again, had no significant effect on these variables.

The mean rate of weight gain during pregnancy in the HIV-positive women was reported in 2002.[19] During the third trimester of pregnancy, average weight gain was significantly greater (by 304g) and the risk of low rate of weight gain (less than or equal to 100g/week) was significantly lower in women who received multivitamins than in women who did not.

Thus, multivitamins not only delayed disease progression and death among HIV-positive pregnant women, but they also improved the survival rates and weight gain of the fetus and the survival prospects of the infant at birth.

The relationship between dietary and supplemental micronutrient intake and subsequent mortality was examined in 281 HIV-infected participants at the Baltimore, Maryland/Washington, DC, site of the Multicenter Acquired Immunodeficiency Syndrome Cohort Study, over an eight-year follow-up period.[20] The highest intake for each B-group vitamin—B_1, B_2, B_6, and niacin—was independently associated with improved survival. Beta-carotene intake at moderately high levels was also associated with improved survival, whereas increasing intake of zinc was associated with poorer survival. Intake of B_6 supplements at more than twice the recommended dietary allowance was associated with improved survival, whereas intake of B_1 and B_2 supplements at levels greater than five times the recommended dietary allowance was associated with improved survival. Any intake of zinc supplements, however, was associated with poorer survival.

In a study of 119 HIV-infected patients, vitamin D intake increased the CD4 cell count at the rate of $34/\mu l$ for each microgram of vitamin D.[21]

A number of other studies showed positive trends toward delaying disease progression in HIV-positive subjects, but their results were not statistically significant. One promising approach is to augment through selenium the level of antioxidants that are often found to be deficient in people with AIDS disease. This is dealt with in detail in the chapter "Selenium Conquers AIDS."

There have been no formal clinical trials on the effect of probiotics on AIDS disease progression, although HIV-positive individuals have taken the initiative to help themselves (see "Probiotics for Life After HIV/AIDS").

Selenium Conquers AIDS

IS **AIDS** LINKED TO SELENIUM DEPLETION?
AND CAN SELENIUM SUPPLEMENTATION CONQUER **AIDS**?

GEOGRAPHIC CLUE TO SELENIUM

During the last decade, research has indicated an important geographical link between regions of selenium-deficient soils and peak incidences of HIV/AIDS infection.[1] AIDS disease appears to involve a slow and progressive decline in levels of the trace element selenium in the blood along with CD4 cells, which are both independent predictors of mortality.[2]

AIDS infection in Africa has reached pandemic proportions, with over a quarter of the population said to be suffering from the disease in some areas, although there is debate over the WHO statistics (see the chapter "The African AIDS Epidemic"). Figures from Harvard put infection rates as follows: Zimbabwe 25.84 percent, Botswana 25.10 percent, Zambia 19.07 percent, South Africa 12.91 percent, Côte D'Ivoire 10.06 percent, Tanzania 9.42 percent, Ethiopia 9.31 percent, and Congo 4.31 percent.

But Senegal in West Africa has the lowest AIDS prevalence at 1.77 percent in the general population, and 0.5 percent in antenatal clinic attendees, along with the most highly selenium-enriched soil.[3] Geologically, Senegal is situated in the dried-up Cretaceous and early Eocene Sea, and the land is formed from sedimentary rocks from dissolved minerals in the evaporating seawater. Consequently, calcium phosphates derived from the selenium-rich phosphorite are one of the country's mined mineral products used for fertilizers. Senegal can also claim the lowest level of cancers on the African continent.[4]

Geographical disease pattern analogies made by Prof. E. W. Taylor, University of Georgia, suggest that AIDS, Kaposi's sarcoma, and cancers are rife in regions of selenium-depleted soils and that this has further implications in the seemingly unstoppable spread of AIDS incidence worldwide.

DEPLETED SELENIUM IN SOIL CREATES DISEASE

In China, selenium-deficient regions are known as the "disease belt." Here, the average daily intake of selenium is less than 10 micrograms. This contrasts with parts of the United States and Canada, where daily selenium intake is 170 micrograms. Viral diseases such as coxsackie B3, hepatitis B and C, and HIV/AIDS are all on the increase. Coxsackie B3 is further complicated by a heart condition known as keshans, which is endemic in the disease belt areas. Since the introduction of selenium-enriched fertilizers onto soils and crops and of selenium into feedstocks and table salt, however, there has been a decline in keshans.

A three-year study of an entire town in Jiangsu Province where 20,847 residents were given table salt fortified with selenium showed that hepatitis infection decreased to 4.52 cases per 1,000 people, compared to 10.48 per 1,000 people in communities using regular table salt.[5] The same researchers concluded that a 200 microgram daily dose of selenium-yeast supplement significantly reduced primary liver cancer associated with hepatitis B and C. It appears that death rates from viruses such as hepatitis, coxsackie B3, and associated heart diseases like keshans can be greatly reduced by increasing dietary selenium intake and would be similarly effective in slowing the progress of AIDS deaths.

THE SELENIUM CD4 T-CELL TAILSPIN

Prof. Harold Foster of the University of Victoria in Canada has named the link between the viral diseases of HIV/AIDS, coxsackie, and hepatitis B and C "the selenium CD4 T-cell tailspin" as a way of describing the relationship between selenium and the human immune system. Adults and children with advanced AIDS syndrome display both highly depleted selenium plasma stores and reduced CD4 cell counts. Foster argues that the fall of selenium levels triggers the reduction in CD4 cells, which in turn causes further decline in serum selenium.[6]

Retroviruses like HIV depress selenium levels in their hosts by encoding the gene for the selanonenzyme (an enzyme dependent on selenium as co-factor) glutathione peroxidase. This allows the virus to replicate indefinitely by continuously depriving the host of glutathione (GSH), an essential antioxidant for the host immune system (see the chapters "Vaccinating People Against Their Own Genes," "Eating Well for Health," and "Eating Well Against HIV/AIDS") and the four basic components of glutathione peroxidase: selenium, cysteine, glutamine, and tryptophan.[7] As levels of selenium decline, so do CD4 cells, which allows opportunistic pathogens to invade the immune system and further deplete the levels of selenium and CD4 cells in a positive feedback loop, whereby if one variable declines, it causes further depression in the others. This downward spiral compromises the ability of the immune system to defend the body from infection, which plays a significant role in AIDS mortality.

Foster is currently treating dozens of HIV/AIDS patients in Africa using a protocol of the four nutrients—selenium, cysteine, glutamine, and tryptophan. He says that the treatment of HIV/AIDS with nutrition is similar to "curing" type 1 diabetes with insulin. When high doses of all four nutrients are administered to patients, deficiencies dissolve, as do the symptoms associated with AIDS. Patients have been able to return to work within one month of receiving nutritional treatments. Treating primary nutritional deficiencies with selenium and essential amino acids costs approximately $10 to $15 (see box).

As HIV/AIDS sufferers are often extremely deficient in all four nutrients associated with glutathione peroxidase, the "selenium CD4 T-cell tailspin" hypothesis, which describes HIV/AIDS as a disease of nutrient deficiency caused by a virus, may explain how HIV progresses to AIDS.

Dr. Roberto Giraldo, president of Rethinking AIDS: The International Group for the Scientific Reappraisal of AIDS, said at a recent seminar in South Africa that AIDS can presently be conquered and curtailed, although not totally cured, through the adequate ingestion of appropriate micronutrients, such as vitamins, amino acids and minerals, in sufficiently large doses.[8]

Four Essential Nutrients

For a healthy person, a daily supplementary intake of 50 to 200 micrograms of selenium is safe, but for someone with a compromised immune system, an increase of 100 percent may be necessary to improve selenium plasma levels. Where soil quality is good and produce fresh, the four essential nutrients in preventing and fighting HIV/AIDS and other viral diseases are found in these foods:

Selenium—Brazil nuts, garlic, mushrooms, liver, round steak, lobster, shrimp, cod, crab, herring, oysters, tuna, barley, whole wheat, egg noodles, brewers yeast

Cysteine—duck, turkey, pork, wheat germ, yogurt

Glutamine—sausage meats, ham, bacon, cottage and ricotta cheeses, wheat germ

Tryptophan—ham, beef, eggs, almonds, salted anchovies, Parmesan and Swiss cheeses

---

The cause of progression of HIV to AIDS is still unknown, but the role of good nutrition and supplements in preventing and treating the disease cannot be ignored. Prof. Luc Montagnier (the co-discoverer of HIV) states that AIDS is characterized by a persistent oxidative imbalance and a decrease of glutathione. Changes in biochemical markers cause systemic oxidative stress and damage, and Montagnier believes that antioxidants are useful in inhibiting viral replication and associated apoptosis (cell death programmed by the body) in HIV/AIDS patients.

THE ROLE OF N-ACETYL CYSTEINE IN BOOSTING IMMUNITY

Glutathione (GSH) is the ubiquitous antioxidant essential for the function of all cells. Studies show that low GSH levels increase HIV replication and impair T-cell function, which can lead to a progression of HIV disease. Oral administration of the GSH-producing drug N-acetyl cysteine (NAC) improves survival rates in HIV/AIDS patients. NAC helps the body synthesize glutathione and is beneficial in protecting lung tissue through its antioxidant activity; it also supports nerve cells and is effective in treating liver failure caused by drug toxicity. NAC also counteracts apoptosis and helps maintain and replenish the HIV-damaged CD4 T-lymphocytes, which is crucial for dampening the progression of HIV to AIDS.[9]

NAC supplement is recommended for HIV/AIDS sufferers, whether or not they are receiving antiretroviral treatments. There is growing evidence that while HIV/AIDS patients want alternative and nontoxic immune-boosting treatments, they would prefer them to be prescribed by doctors or health care professionals. Despite billions of dollars spent on AIDS research, pharmaceutical drugs hold a virtual monopoly on AIDS treatment in the United States and Canada.[10] Similarly, very little funding or research is allocated for the provision of alternative treatments on the National Health Service in the U.K.[11]

Raising glutathione levels encourages the immune system to go into anticancer and antiviral mode by replacing decreased levels of plasma cysteine, a major source of sulfur. Patients with advanced HIV infection have tryptophan levels at less than 50 percent of those in age- and gender-matched controls; boosting levels of the amino acid tryptophan can enable the body to synthesize serotonin and niacin, which protect against dementia. Improving glutamine levels can alleviate depression and improve digestion by increasing intestinal cell proliferation and intestinal fluid/electrolyte absorption, which can help combat diarrhea.[12]

THE CAUSE OF SELENIUM DEPLETION IN SOIL

Three major factors have contributed to selenium depletion in the soil. Acid rain is caused by large quantities of sulfur and nitrogen that convert into sulfuric and nitric acids in the atmosphere, and this changes the pH of the soil and its capacity to bind elements. The altered pH balance increases bioavailability of certain elements and decreases that of others, including selenium. Heavy metals in rainfall also contain mercury, which can combine with selenium to produce the insoluble mercury selenide. Soil acidification therefore lowers the abundance of selenium in the global food chain, which may have contributed to the rapid increase of cancers and HIV/AIDS.[13]

Chlorofluorocarbons are unique to the latter half of the twentieth century and have contributed to the thinning of the ozone layer, which causes an excess of ultraviolet-B radiation. Overexposure to ultraviolet light decreases helper T-lymphocytes and increases suppressor T-lymphocytes, making the individual more susceptible to diseases.[14]

Chemical pollutants also play a role in altering the immune function and lowering host resistance to pathogens. WHO estimates that there are 500,000 pesticide-related illnesses and 20,000 pesticide-related deaths per year. Scientific studies show that polychlorinated biphenyls (PCBs) depress glutathione peroxidase activity and induce apoptosis of pre–B-lymphocytes in the plasma of animals.[15]

Whey protein, a derivative of milk production routinely discarded by the dairy industry, contains all the essential and nonessential amino acids necessary to improve immunity by increasing glutathione levels in the blood.[16] Oral supplement of whey proteins can also help combat wasting associated with AIDS.

A wide variety of nutrients, vitamins, amino acids, herbs, and minerals such as copper, zinc, and selenium are clearly beneficial in slowing death rates in HIV-infected individuals[17] (see the chapter "Eating Well Against HIV/AIDS"). And vitamins A, C, and E can help reduce the oxidative stress and viral load that characterize HIV/AIDS sufferers.[18] This is especially important in areas where combination therapies are unavailable.

And yet, in Europe, moves are afoot to prohibit the sale of fourteen forms of organic selenium supplement, selenium yeast, and selenomethionine if the E.U. Directive on Food Supplements comes into force in August 2005.[19] This must be rigorously challenged as unethical and detrimental to the health of people suffering from life-threatening diseases like AIDS.

Probiotics for Life
After HIV/AIDS

PROBIOTICS HAVE BEEN ENLISTED IN THE FIGHT AGAINST **HIV/AIDS.**

PROBIOTICS WORK

Sandor Ellix Katz, a long-term AIDS survivor, calls himself a "fermentation fetishist," being very impressed with the healing effects of live cultured foods. He is spreading the message in his new book, *Wild Fermentation: The Flavour, Nutrition and Craft of Live-culture Foods.*[1]

The book is strongly recommended by Rebecca Wood, a great advocate for the healing power of food as medicine and the power of fermented food to strengthen the immune system.[2] Wood claims to have cured herself of advanced cervical cancer fifteen years ago through a healing diet. She says that she has helped many others since through her books and her Web site (see the end of this chapter for the Web address).

She points out that fermented foods are found in every traditional cuisine, where natural enzymes, fungi, and bacteria predigest vegetable, fruit, or animal products, increasing their flavor and their nutritional and medicinal value. Live-cultured foods, especially those high in lactic acid, strengthen the immune system by maintaining a healthy population of microflora in the gut.

The healthy adult gastrointestinal tract contains over two pounds of microflora that can be destroyed by antibiotics, antibiotic residues contained in commercial meats, chlorinated water, spirits, and a highly processed diet heavy in sugar, salt, and non–cold-pressed vegetable oils.

Unprocessed fermented foods boost the immune system by aiding digestion and increasing antibodies that fight infectious disease. The flora in living cultured foods form a shield that covers the small intestine's inner lining and helps inhibit pathogenic organisms such as *Candida albicans* (yeast).

Some fermented foods create antioxidants (glutathione and superoxide dismutase) which scavenge free radicals that may cause cancer.

Fermenting transforms milk-sugar lactose—which most adult animals, including the vast majority of adult humans, cannot digest—to the metabolite lactic acid. Lactic acid also neutralizes the antinutrients found in many foods.

Fermentation generates B vitamins and new nutrients including essential omega-3 fatty acids, digestive aids, and the trace mineral GTF (glucose tolerance factor) chromium, which plays a role in regulating blood sugar levels. These vitamins and nutrients are vital to good health.

Many probiotic bacteria, such as *Lactobacillus acidophilus* and *L. bifidus*, can be found in yogurt and buttermilk with active cultures. Other tasty choices include kefir (a fermented dairy product containing thirty different strains of beneficial microorganisms), miso (a fermented soybean seasoning agent), sauerkraut (pickled cabbage), and a pickled Korean cabbage called kimchee.

DETOXIFYING THE GUT

Detoxifying the gut is a prerequisite to rebuilding the immune system, according to Roberto Giraldo, a medical doctor and president of Rethinking AIDS: The International Group for the Scientific Reappraisal of AIDS.[3] Mark Konlee, author of *The Immune Restoration Handbook*, which has sold nearly 2 million copies, agrees.

Konlee has promoted cutting-edge information on issues relating to immune-compromised conditions such as HIV/AIDS based on both scientific research and anecdotal evidence since 1994. He has reached, helped, and empowered many individuals via his Web site (see the end of this chapter for the Web address).

Konlee says, "Having a preponderance of friendly bacteria in the colon is not an option for healthy intestines, it is a requirement." The food choices we make daily determine whether health-promoting or disease-promoting flora prevail in our bodies.[4]

Probiotic *Bifidobacterium* species, reintroduced into the gastrointestinal tract, produce butyric acid that helps rebuild the mucous membranes and heal the leaks in the unhealthy gut. They also produce proprionic acid and acetic acid (as found in vinegar) that kill pathogens and aid the absorption of calcium, magnesium, iron, and many trace elements vital to endocrine and hormonal balance. These acidic products of friendly bacteria also lower the pH of the colon.

Research has shown that pathogens thrive in an alkaline environment above pH 7, and HIV loses the ability to infect CD4 cells below a pH of 6. The gut's acidic environment is further augmented by the production of lactic acid by *Lactobacillus* species. These acids, which deter the replication of HIV, are short-chain fatty acids that make the stools lighter than water, so that they float. Large-diameter, golden-brown, floating stools are said to be the sign of a healthy gut.[5] Friendly flora also produce B vitamins that turn urine yellow.[6]

The small and large intestines, therefore, need to be supplemented with probiotics sufficient to destroy toxins, heal mucous membranes, and create a stable, healthy, more acidic environment. Foods that promote probiotics include fructo-oligosaccharides (FOSs), which reach the lower intestines intact and are devoured there by *B. longum*, *L. bifidus*, and other friendly bacteria, allowing them to flourish. Fructo-oligosaccharides can be taken in their natural form as artichokes, chicory, whole rye, bananas, onions, garlic, and asparagus.[7]

STRENGTHENING THE IMMUNE SYSTEM

Probiotic microflora colonize the gut, which has 200 times more surface area than the skin, and where about half the body's immune cells are activated to protect the interior of the body from harmful material.[8] HIV prefers to infect these activated cells and thrives in the gut lymphoid tissue, even when minimal viral activity is demonstrated in the blood.[9]

These microflora also help balance the two arms of the immune system, cell-mediated and humoral immunity (see "Vaccinating People Against Their Own Genes").

The disease-ridden environment of the unhealthy gut causes leaks in the structure of the epithelium, through which byproducts of faulty digestion enter the blood and trigger an antibody response (Th2). This systematically weakens the cell-mediated immune response (Th1).[10]

As HIV infection progresses from the asymptomatic phase to advanced disease, the immune response appears to shift from the failing Th1 to the overstimulated Th2 state. Restoring and balancing these two interdependent arms of the immune system could protect against many chronic illnesses such as AIDS[11].

Restoring the mucous membranes of the gastrointestinal tract as the natural barrier that prevents invasion by pathogenic viruses, bacteria, fungi, and so forth is therefore essential. Restoring normal Th1 cytokines, especially IL-12, which stimulates a CD8 killer T-cell response, and IFN-γ and IgA, which give mucosal immunity, are critical first steps.

PROBIOTICS ARE FOR LIFE

High levels of Th1 cytokines have been found repeatedly in the mucous membranes of long-term HIV/AIDS survivors.[12] Strengthening these Th1 cytokines requires the patient to eat fresh, healthful food slowly, mixing it with saliva, and only when hungry. Probiotics *Lactobacillus plantarum* and *L. casei* are exceptional stimulators of Th1 cytokines. They induce a strong IL-12 response and increase IFN-g and the systemic immune response against all intracellular viral infections. *Lactobacillus casei* has also been found to suppress IL-4, -5, -6, and -10 (Th2 cytokines). *Bifidobacterium longum* has been found to increase IgA and improve mucosal immunity (Th1 response).[13]

A calcium-supplemented diet has been found to increase *L. acidophilus* growth and strongly increase the resistance to *Salmonella enteritidis* in the small intestines of experimental rats.[14] High-calcium foods that support the growth of *L. acidophilus* and offer excellent nutrition include collard greens, dandelion greens, beet greens, mustard greens, turnip greens, parsley, kale, spinach, watercress, and endive. Live dairy products, fish, kelp, seaweed, spirulina, blue-green algae, and blackstrap molasses are excellent. Tofu, carrots, squash, pumpkin, buckwheat, cabbage, wheatgrass, barley, and rye are also good for calcium and minerals.[15]

More information on probiotics, nutrition, and diet regimes can be found at the Web sites of Sandor Ellix Katz (www.wildfermentation.com) and Rebecca Wood (www.rwood.com). Mark Konlee publishes the quarterly *Journal of Immunity*, available online at www.keephopealive.org.

Herbs for Immunity

TRADITIONAL MEDICINAL PLANTS AND THEIR SUGAR
MOLECULES ARE EFFECTIVE IMMUNE SYSTEM BOOSTERS.

IMMUNITY COMES INTO FOCUS

Since the onset of what has now become the global phenomenon of HIV/AIDS, the immune system has come under the spotlight of "whole body healing" or holistic healing. The individual's immune system is a barometer of how the person is feeling: whether stressed, run down, tired, or depressed. Good health simply reflects a balanced physiological state of security against disease.

Just before birth and thereafter, an individual progressively acquires specific immunity as B- (bone) lymphocytes and T- (thymus) lymphocytes, the backbone of humoral and cellular immunity, become activated by antigens. Immunity is built over time as infants grow through adolescence into adulthood and then declines in old age. Two of the most vulnerable groups in society—children and the elderly—have immune systems that are either not fully developed or are in decline.[1]

Similarly, people living with HIV/AIDS are vulnerable members of the community who have special needs in regard to boosting their immunity. But the cocktails of conventional antiretroviral therapies prescribed to treat disease destroy many healthy cells in the process as the body attempts to respond to the drugs with an increasingly compromised immune system.[2]

TRADITIONAL VS. CONVENTIONAL MEDICINE

Many conventional cancer treatments succeed and the patient makes a full recovery, but for the others, chemical treatments on top of the disease overwhelm the body's defenses. This stark reality has led many with life-threatening illnesses like cancer and HIV/AIDS to use alternative medicines in addition to or instead of conventional medicine to give their bodies a fighting chance of survival.[3]

Herbal medicine is no different from conventional medicine when it is considered only in terms of blood and T- and B-cells, but the human immune system may also be viewed as an interface between individuals and their world.[4] The new physics of the organism and the complexity of the "fluid genome" suggest that life is a dynamic dance in which all parts of the organism are constantly seeking harmony simultaneously within and with the rest of nature.[5] The immune system, therefore, plays a major role in integrating the individual into society and the broader ecosystem.

Holistic or traditional healing methods like herbalism, ayurveda, and homeopathy are the closest systems that we have to "customized" medicine designed to suit the individual, something that geneticists aspire to develop. This is because herbal medicine addresses all aspects of human life. Holistic healing involves ensuring that the body receives the correct nutrition and the appropriate therapy to address any illness that may be present. The emotional health of the patient is also nurtured; the individual's likes and dislikes, thoughts and feelings, and hopes and fears are all considered when prescribing any course of treatment.

Herbal medicine as an ecological medicine is starting to make sense in terms of the geographical distribution of HIV/AIDS associated with areas of selenium depletion (see the chapter "Selenium Conquers AIDS"). It is of considerable interest that an indigenous plant essential for treating appetite loss and AIDS-associated wasting grows bountifully in areas of South Africa where HIV infection is estimated at 6 million, as will be described in the next chapter.

In the West there has been little effort to integrate complementary and alternative medicine (CAM) into healthcare systems (see Table 1); more funding and political will is needed to do this.[6]

Table 1. Use of Traditional Medicine Worldwide

Estimated Use of TM /CAM Worldwide	Healthcare System Integration of TM/CAM	Cost Estimates of TM/CAM Worldwide
Africa	Used by 80% as primary healthcare	
China	30%–50% of total consumption; fully integrated; 95% hospitals have units for TM	
India	Widely used; 2,860 hospitals provide TM	
Indonesia	Used by 40% of overall population, 70% of rural population	
Japan	72% of MDs practice TM	
Thailand	TM integrated into 1,120 health centers	
Vietnam	Fully integrated into healthcare system; 30% of population treated with TM	
Western countries	TM/CAM not integrated into healthcare systems	
U.S.A.	40% of population uses CAM	
France	75% have used CAM at least once	
Germany	77% of pain clinics provide acupuncture	
Australia		$1 billion
China (herbal)		$1.8 billion
Japan (herbal)		$1.4 billion
U.K.		$2.3 billion
U.S.A.		$27 billion
Global		$60 billion

Source: WHO factsheet no. 271, June 2002

Activation of the immune system can be achieved on several levels with single remedies or combinations of herbs with synergistic effects. Strengthening and supporting the whole physiological system is the herbalist's goal, rather than specifically stimulating or inhibiting different molecular or cellular components of the immune system. Phytochemicals that can affect human tissue are known as *deep immune activators*. Remedies that work on the hormones are called *adaptogens*, and building resistance of the immune system is known as *surface immune activation*.

An increasing number of alternative or traditional medicine protocols exist for treating HIV/AIDS. Some healing herbs that are common to many such systems are described below.

ASTRAGALUS

Astragalus membranaceous or *huang qi* (yellow leader) originates from China and is a highly prized and ancient herbal medicine.[7] Its use as a tonic that strengthens the body and promotes tissue healing has been documented in the *Chinese Herbal Materia Medica* for over four millennia.

The medicinal properties of the sweet, warming root are attributed to a group of carbohydrates: saponins, polysaccharides, and in particular cycloartane glycosides, which are high-weight polymers of monosaccharides containing glucose and other sugars.[8] But one study suggests that isoflavones (nonsteroid estrogens) show potential antiviral activity.[9]

Nutritionists and scientists are examining the role of sugars or glyconutrients on human immunity. Sugars combine with proteins and fats to create glycoform molecules, which coat the surface of virtually every cell in the body. Of the eight simple sugars (see Table 2), many are missing from the standard modern diet, which contributes to a breakdown in cell communication. A glyconutrient (GN) supplement comprising various polysaccharides is listed in the *U.S. Physicians Desk Reference of Nonprescription Drugs and Dietary Supplements*. GN is documented to powerfully stimulate the macrophages, which in turn orchestrate the activity of the other cells, including natural killer (NK) cells.[10]

Table 2. Eight Simple Sugars and Their Food Sources

Sugar	Food Source
Mannose	Aloe vera; shiitake mushrooms; kelp; ground fenugreek
Glucose	Abundant in diet, especially honey and bee products; grapes, bananas, mangoes, cherries, strawberries; licorice, hawthorn, garlic, sarsaparilla, cocoa
Galactose	Apples, apricots, bananas, cranberries, currants, dates, peaches; soybeans; avocado, capsicum (cayenne), cabbage, celery, eggplant, tomato, turnip, pumpkin, green beans
Fucose	Seaweed—kelp, wakame; beer yeast
N-acetylglucoasamine	Bovine cartilage, shark cartilage; shiitake mushrooms
N-acetylgalactosamine	Bovine cartilage, shark cartilage; a red algae called *Dumontiaceae* (a constituent of dextran sulfate, available only in Japan)
Xylose 1 and xylose 2	Guava, pears, blackberries, loganberries, raspberries; aloe vera, *Echinacea*; *Psyllium* seeds; broccoli, spinach, okra, corn, peas
N-acetylneuraminic acid	Whey protein isolate; hen's eggs

Modern herbalists use *Astragalus* as an immune-boosting tonic, often combined with other herbs such as ginseng and licorice, but no human trials have been conducted to assess the benefits of *Astragalus* on HIV patients. *In vitro* trials show that *Astragalus* extracts enhance immune activity and induce lymphokine-activated killer-cell activity in cancer and HIV patients.[11]

Astragalus extract also markedly stimulates normal cells to proliferate; it enhances the activation of mononuclear cells and macrophages and the production of cytokines, tumor necrosis factor, and IL-6; but it has no influence on natural killer cells.[12]

GINSENG

Siberian ginseng (*Eleuthroccus senticosus*), American ginseng (*Panax quin-quefolius*), and Asian ginseng (*P. ginseng*) are all members of the Araliaceae family and native to Asia, China, and Russia.

In Russia, HIV infection was estimated to be at 700,000 in 2001, with 3,623 officially registered cases. By 2004, 1,400,000 cases were estimated and 284,914 cases registered

In China, HIV was first reported in 1985; by 2001, 28,133 cases were registered as HIV-positive, with 1,208 AIDS cases and 641 AIDS deaths.[13] In 2004 an estimated 1,313,309 people were living with HIV/AIDS. There had been a 90 percent increase in infection in Chinese sex workers in the Guangxi region. Forty percent of the global total of persons with HIV/AIDS live in Asia,[14] so it is crucially important to draw on indigenous herbal treatments that are readily available.

An adaptogen tonic (a substance that invigorates and strengthens the body) made from the three distinct species of ginseng is traditionally used to treat weakness and fatigue in Asia. More recently, it has been used to treat a variety of diseases, including cancer.[15] The history of ginseng goes back thousands of years; the literal translation of *Panax* is "cure-all." *P. ginseng* has proved effective as an immune system booster and significantly improves physical performance during exercise.[16,17] Exercise plays an important role in maintaining health and preventing disease, but it can also significantly improve the health of HIV/AIDS patients (see the chapter "Exercise Versus AIDS").

Ginseng's active agents include triterpene saponins, polysaccharides, and ginsenosides, thirty-one of which have been isolated from white and red ginseng. They reside in the slow-growing roots, which can live up to 100 years. It is thought that ginseng affects the functions of the hypothalamus-pituitary-adrenal axis (endocrine system) and in turn the immune system. Studies on animals and *in vitro* tests on human tissue have shown that *P. ginseng* enhances phagocytosis, natural killer-cell activity, and the production of interferon. At the University of Milan, studies showed that *P. ginseng* increased all cell-mediated immune parameters, including T-lymphocytes (T3) and T-helper cells (T4). Total lymphocyte count and T-cell production were also increased over an eight-week regimen of a standardized ginseng preparation.[18]

Ginseng has many uses, but dwindling wild stocks mean that more cultivated products are on the market. Japanese scientists have observed the difference in immune effects between wild and cultured *P. ginseng*.[19] Mice given extracts of wild ginseng showed a greater increase of T-cells and T-helper cells than mice given extracts of cultured ginseng.

ALOE VERA

Aloe vera (*Aloe vulgaris* or *A. barbadensis*) is a succulent plant belonging to the lily family (Liliaceae), with perennial strong and fibrous roots and abundant fleshy leaves edged with spiny teeth. Aloe vera consists of very large mucosaccharides. The most important long-chain sugars are those containing mannose and glucose, as well as twenty polysaccharides and twenty-three polypeptides that help control a broad spectrum of immune system diseases and immune disorders.

A mannose-containing mucopolysaccharide has been extracted from the plant and patented under the name of acemannan. A double-blind trial was conducted of its effect on patients with HIV. An oral daily dose of 1,600mg of acemannan did not prevent decline in CD4 counts. Acemannan showed no significant effect on p24 antigen or amount of virus in the bloodstream. Acemannan did not cause side effects or interact negatively with AZT.[20]

A team of scientists led by Dr. Terry Pulse used mucopolysaccharides orally with good results. Patients improved clinically and functionally; 93.1 percent of the patients showed an improvement on the Karnofsky scale (commonly used to assess terminally ill patients) at 90 days, and 100 percent at 180 days. In 51.7 percent of patients, T4-helper lymphocytes increased at 90 days and in 32.2 percent at 180 days, with 25 percent reactive HIV p24 core antigen converted to negative at 90 days and 180 days. Patients reported that within three to five days, their energy levels improved, lymph nodes decreased in size, coughs improved, diarrhea stopped, and they gained weight. AZT-induced anemia was improved on the regime of Aloe vera juice; opportunistic infections ceased; and patients were able to return to normal activity.[21]

Aloe's mucopolysaccharides are derived from the mucilage layers of the plant that encase the inner gel. When ingested, the mucopolysaccharides are phagocytized by macrophages, which release cytokines that activate interleukins and lymphocytes to attack their targets (see "Vaccinating People Against Their Own Genes"). Mucopolysaccharides and polysaccharides are not broken down like other sugars but remain undigested, appearing in the bloodstream in the same form, where they exert their immune regulation by being taken up into cells in a soluble form.

Scientists from Texas A&M University say that a complex carbohydrate compound purified from the aloe vera plant appears to help drugs such as AZT and acyclovir block the pathology associated with HIV and herpes simplex virus. They also found that the compound interfered with HIV's ability to reproduce in infected cells. Dr. Maurice Kemp, a virologist in Texas, notes: "It's not going to be a magic bullet against AIDS, there aren't many magic bullets out there. But as an adjunctive therapy, it looks like it can be used in combination with other therapies."[22]

OLIVE LEAF

The olive leaf is a symbol of peace and has been around since the writing of the Book of Genesis. Olive leaf contains a phenolic glucoside called oleuropein, which has powerful antiviral properties.[23] Its use as an alternative protease inhibitor was recognized by the AIDS community in 1996. Olive leaf also has anti–RT ability and selectively kills virus cells without harming human DNA polymerase. This is due to the presence of calcium elenolate, a chemical compound derived from oleuropein, which has been found to inactivate many viruses tested against it.[24]

Olive leaf extract has been used in combination with conventional drugs.[25] Naltrexone is an immune-stabilizing drug that can stop the progression of AIDS disease and a decline in the immune system by regulating key hormones and improving communication between the brain and the immune function. It is usually used to help drug- and alcohol-dependent patients. No side effects have been reported.

Olive leaf extract can also be combined with lemon juice for a variation of the treatment. This remedy appears to be helpful in reversing swollen lymph nodes, wasting syndrome, and neuropathy. Mark Konlee, editor of *Positive Health News*, has reported some encouraging anecdotal evidence using this protocol (see www.keephope.net).

LICORICE

Licorice (*Glycyrrhiza glabra*) roots are unearthed in the autumn and have been traditionally used as a treatment for coughs and bronchial problems. Licorice's sweet-tasting triterpenoid saponin is glycyrrhizin (a glycoside), one of several members of a chemical group called sulfated polysaccharides that have demonstrated varying degrees of anti-HIV activity.

A study of twenty asymptomatic HIV-positive patients at Osaka National Hospital, Japan, was reported at the Fifth International Conference on AIDS in Montreal in 1989.[26] Ten patients were given daily oral doses of glycyrrhizin ranging from 150 to 225mg, and none progressed to symptoms over periods of one to two years. In the control group of ten who were not treated, one developed swollen lymph glands and two others were diagnosed with AIDS and subsequently died.

Another study was sponsored in Japan by Tohoku University, Fukushima Medical College, and Akita University. Nine patients with hemophilia who were HIV-positive but asymptomatic were given 200 to 800mg of intravenous glycyrrhizin daily for over eight weeks. Eight patients experienced an average 88.9 percent increase in T4-helper cells, and six experienced an average 66.7 percent improvement in their T4/T8 ratio. Liver dysfunction noted in four patients improved, and no serious side effects were observed.[27] Licorice also contains coumarins and flavonoids, compounds that are helpful antioxidants. Glycyrrhizin is available over the counter in Japan at a cost of 10 cents per 25 g pill.

MANY PROMISING HERBS FOR IMMUNITY

The traditional herbal medicines that might improve immunity against HIV/AIDS are too many to list. Other promising candidates include neem extracts and guaifenesin,[28] garlic,[29–33] propolis,[33–35] and milk thistle.[36]

In the next few chapters, we shall describe work done with specific herbs and extracts in more detail.

Traditional Medicine in the Fight Against AIDS

WHILE BILLIONS OF DOLLARS HAVE BEEN PLEDGED TO HELP THE WORST AFFECTED, MANY OF THE POOREST COUNTRIES ARE STILL LEFT WITHOUT THE MEDICAL SUPPORT AVAILABLE IN THE WEST, AND UP TO 80 PERCENT OF THE POPULATION MUST RELY ON TRADITIONAL MEDICINE FOR PRIMARY HEALTHCARE.

MEDICINAL HERBS OF GREAT HEALING TRADITIONS

Medicinal plants have been part of the great healing traditions around the world going back thousands of years, the best known being the Indian ayurvedic medical system, traditional Chinese medicine, and Western herbal medicine. These traditional medicines are the basis of a quarter of all drugs in today's modern pharmacy.[1]

WHO defines traditional medicine as health practices, approaches, knowledge, and beliefs incorporating plant-, animal-, and mineral-based medicines, spiritual therapies, and manual techniques (e.g., reflexology) applied singularly or in combination to treat, diagnose, and prevent illness or maintain well-being. In 2002, WHO launched its first comprehensive traditional medicine strategy to assist efforts to promote affordable, effective, and safe use of traditional medicine (TM) and complementary alternative medicine (CAM).[2]

In Africa, TM is used by up to 80 percent of the population to meet primary healthcare needs and is crucial in the fight against infectious diseases. The ratio of conventional, or Western-trained, general practitioners to patients is 1:20,000, whereas the availability of TM practitioners is 1:200 to 1:400. This highlights the need for reliable and affordable herbal medicines that are locally available.[3]

In South Africa, it is estimated that over 6 million people are living with HIV/AIDS, and 150 babies are born with HIV every day. Conventional drugs exist for the treatment of HIV/AIDS, but they are only affordable by an estimated 1 percent of sufferers.

RELIANCE ON TRADITIONAL MEDICINE IN TREATING AIDS

Three of four AIDS patients in Africa rely on some form of TM for treating the symptoms of HIV/AIDS. A wide range of traditional herbal medicine is used (see Table 3). One of them, *Sutherlandia*, has emerged as a major treatment for AIDS.

Sutherlandia frutescens (subspecies *microphylla*) belongs to Fabaceae, a subfamily of Leguminosae (peas and beans). It is a perennial shrub that grows wild in the arid regions of Botswana, Namibia, Zululand, and the Western and Eastern Cape regions of Africa. *Sutherlandia* can grow to a little over one-and-a-half yards in height in optimum conditions of stony grasslands exposed to constant sunshine in daylight hours. Blood-red flowers bloom from June to December, and seeds are carried in greenish-red papery pods, which are almost transparent. The compound pinnate leaves have a green-gray color, giving the bush a silvery appearance.[4]

The leaves and branches of the *Sutherlandia* bush are bitter to the taste but are thought traditionally to have health-giving properties. The dried leaves, containing four active compounds, are ground by traditional healers to make into tonics, teas, pills, or creams (see Table 3). In the absence of easily available and affordable antiretrovirals, these herbal treatments are used as the first line of defense in combating the symptoms of AIDS and other wasting diseases. Practitioners of traditional medicine who prescribe *Sutherlandia* are keen to preserve the use of the plant as a traditional remedy to maintain its patent-free status.

Table 3. Patient Symptoms and Traditional Medicines Prescribed at Ngwelezane Hospital, South Africa

Primary Symptoms	Traditional Medicines
Cough, cold, bronchitis	*Lippia javanica* (*umsuzwane*)—fresh leaves to make tea infusion
Chest pain	*Warburgia salutaris* (*isibaha*)—two fresh leaves in tea infusion; contraindicated in pregnancy
Diarrhea	*Psidium guajava* (guava)—two crushed leaves with plenty of liquid; discontinue when symptoms subside
Itchy, painful rashes	*Centella asiatica* (pennywort)—fresh leaves blended with glycerine to make cream
Fucose	Seaweed—kelp, wakame; beer yeast
Headaches, shortness of breath	*Artemisia afra* (*umhylonyane*)—fresh aromatic leaves inhaled from gauze bag to ease symptoms
Loss of energy, weakness	*Hypoxis hemerocallidea* (*inkomfe*)—weak infusions made from corms of African potato; excellent strengthening tonic, but must be used under medical supervision
Loss of weight/appetite	*Sutherlandia* (*unwele*)—tablets made from dried leaves; 300mg tablet twice a day with meals (half-dose for child)
Oral sores, body sores, swelling	*Bulibine frutescens* (*ibhucu*)—sap from leaves, applied directly or in a cream
Throat infections	*Siphononchilus aethiopicus* (African ginger; *indungulu*)—tablets made from rhizomes derived from fresh roots

Secondary symptoms reported by patients at Ngwelezane Clinic: abdominal pain, night sweats/fevers, urinary problems, nausea/vomiting, and swollen glands. All the above recommended traditional medical treatments were given by healthcare professionals at an HIV/AIDS clinic in Ngwelezane, South Africa.

145

CONVENTIONAL AND TRADITIONAL HEALERS JOIN UP

An independent, interdisciplinary partnership of traditional healers, botanists, conventional doctors, and scientists have formed the group PhytoNova to prescribe and record the medicinal benefits of *Sutherlandia* in the treatment of HIV/AIDS symptoms. The PhytoNova team has shared knowledge and experience of the medicinal benefits of *Sutherlandia*, particularly in the supportive treatment of people living with HIV/AIDS. *Sutherlandia* is used to boost the immune system of such patients, which may delay progression of the disease, and can also be considered by physicians for use with antiretroviral treatments where available, or as an alternative treatment if side effects from conventional medicine are intolerable.

Dr. Nigel Gericke, a general practitioner and botanist, and his colleague Mr. Credo Mutwa, an eighty-two-year-old traditional healer (*sanusi*), lead PhytoNova's clinical practice and laboratory in Cape Town, South Africa.

PhytoNova makes and supplies medicinal remedies derived from cultivated *Sutherlandia*, of a variety specially selected for its plant chemical profile, for the treatment of HIV/AIDS symptoms direct to doctors, nurses, NGOs, and patients in the region. Key information was released into the public domain early on in the development of the product by PhytoNova to prevent important novel activities of the plant from being patented. The plant has the ability to enhance the immune system and, more specifically, to encourage CD4 cell production in immune-compromised patients, as well as profoundly stimulating appetite and anti-wasting activities in wasted patients. This does not prevent patents being taken out on isolated pure chemical constituents of the plant, but open dissemination of information has encouraged other companies to make *Sutherlandia* products available and has generated a great deal of academic research into the plant's many biological activities. It has also encouraged farmers to plant *Sutherlandia* as a crop.

The price to Africans for a month's supply of pills made from the *Sutherlandia* bush is £2.50 ($4.75), and the powder form of the dried leaves, which is thought to be more effective because of its bitter taste, costs less than 60p ($1.14) for a two-month supply.[5]

Gericke describes the promotion of weight gain in wasted patients with full-blown AIDS as *Sutherlandia*'s principal and most valuable medicinal property. Frequent significant and often sustainable gains in weight have been recorded in HIV patients taking *Sutherlandia* tablets.

Weight records of 244 patients receiving *Sutherlandia* treatment between November 1999 and September 2002 are available from the HIV/AIDS clinic at the Ngwelezane Hospital. Weight increases of up to 33 pounds (15kg) were reported in the majority, and in some cases gains of 6.6 to 11 pounds (3 to 5kg) were sustained over the entire record-keeping period.[6] This physiological boost has the immediate effect of enhancing energy levels and improving the patient's mood. Gericke says, "We have seen several examples of bedridden patients able to get up after a month's treatment and even to return to subsistence farming."[7] Other AIDS patients who were told to "go away and die" by their families or the medical establishment are delighted to find themselves still alive three years after being treated by Mutwa. This anecdotal evidence supports the theory that AIDS may have become a chronic illness rather than a fatal one.

Gericke has informed South African government scientists of the benefits of *Sutherlandia*. These include improvements in appetite, weight gain, sleep, exercise tolerance, anxiety, and an overall sense of well-being. But "because it was a tonic, the scientists dismissed it. They always rush, with classical reductionist thinking, to look for the magic ingredient," says Gericke, summing up the reality that HIV/AIDS itself is so complex that it is increasingly apparent there is no "one-stop" solution for its treatment.[8] Gericke has also appealed to his government to grow the bush on a massive scale and to mobilize a public health drive, but these recommendations too were ignored. To protect wild stocks of the plant from overharvesting in the region, he has contracted local farmers to grow acres of *Sutherlandia* shrubs. This precautionary approach has created local employment and maintained the "not at risk" status of *Sutherlandia* as a medicinal plant.

PhytoNova is convinced that progression to AIDS from HIV can be delayed once the patient has agreed to receive the appropriate treatment and doses of *Sutherlandia*, which are taken on an ongoing basis, in addition to careful attention to diet. It is recommended that alcohol, recreational drugs, and other drugs that damage the immune system be avoided. Anne Hutchings, an ethnobotanist and researcher of traditional Zulu medicine at the University of Zululand, who works in the weekly HIV and AIDS clinic at Ngwelezane Hospital, supports these prescriptions. She uses *Sutherlandia*-derived products from PhytoNova in addition to her own remedies made from local plants (see Table 3). She started with just 11 patients in 1999 and now has more than 400.[9]

In 2001, a community-based AIDS hospice in Emoyeni, South Africa, admitted seventy-one AIDS patients for terminal care. Sister Priscilla Dlamini treated the patients with *Sutherlandia* pills and infusions of another local plant often referred to as African potato (*Hypoxis hermero-callidea*). PhytoNova tracked the progress of her patients one year later. Of the seventy-one patients, thirty had been discharged as healthy back into the community. Some have since returned for follow-up treatments with *Sutherlandia*, while others have been lost to follow-up treatments. No adverse events were reported.[10]

Virginia Rathele is a nurse and Zulu traditional healer (*sangoma*) in the Northern Cape town of Kuruman. She is using *Sutherlandia* pills to treat three hundred AIDS patients in her clinic. She says, "*Sutherlandia* does not work properly just on a diet of porridge. You have to have vegetables." One of her adult patients was close to death and weighed only fifty-seven pounds (26kg), but after receiving treatment and an improved diet now weighs ninety-nine pounds (45kg) and is helping run the clinic. Rathele is also anxious to keep the plant patent-free and believes the treatment should be accessible to everyone.

TRADITIONAL MEDICINE "DISPELS THE DARKNESS"

Historically, *Sutherlandia* has been called many names and used for many purposes. The indigenous Koi San tribespeople call it *insiswa*, which means "the one that dispels darkness." *Insiswa* has been used for centuries as an energy booster and antidepressant. *Sangoma*s know the plant as *unwele*, a "great medicine" that so uplifts your spirit that you will not want to tear your hair out. It was prescribed for the widows of Zulu warriors. *Kankerbos*, "cancer bush," is another name given to *Sutherlandia* by Afrikaners that attests to its traditional use as a cancer remedy. *Sutherlandia* came to the attention of British botanists when Zulu *sangoma*s used it against the 1918 influenza pandemic that killed 20 million worldwide. The English version of *Sutherlandia* was named after James Sutherland, the first superintendent of the Edinburgh Botanical Gardens.[11]

Sutherlandia has a "beautiful portfolio of chemicals," says Gericke (see the box below). Professor Ben-Erik van Wyk and Dr. Carl Albrecht of PhytoNova have analyzed and identified a range of known plant chemicals that previously have been known to have potential application in the treatment of patients with cancer, TB, diabetes, schizophrenia, and depression, and as antiretrovirals. Some of these molecules, already identified from sources other than *Sutherlandia*, have U.S. patents attached to them for their use in treatment of these conditions.[12] Gericke recognizes the great potential of the plant's chemistry and says: "The claim we are making on the basis of this, is that we can dramatically improve the quality of life of many AIDS patients. We are certainly not making the absurd claim that *Sutherlandia* is a cure-all or a cure for AIDS."[13]

The medical records of a patient who had ceased taking conventional antiretrovirals to combat symptoms of HIV/AIDS for two years before turning to PhytoNova for treatments using *Sutherlandia* pills show a marked decrease in the patient's viral load and a significant increase of his CD4 lymphocyte cell count over a six-week period. His starting CD4 count in May 2001 was 340, which increased to 647 in June 2001. During the same period his viral load decreased from 25,000 to 9,200.[14]

Medicinal Compounds Isolated from the Leaves of *Sutherlandia frutescens* (subspecies *microphylla*)

L-canavanine is a potent nonprotein amino acid, l-arginine antagonist with documented antiviral, antibacterial, antifungal, and anticancer activities. L-canavanine has patented antiviral activity against influenza and retrovirus, including HIV. A U.S. patent registered in 1988 claims selective destruction of 95 percent of HIV-infected lymphocytes *in vitro*.

Pinitol is a known antidiabetic agent, described in its 1996 patent as having some benefits in the clinical application of treating wasting in cancer and HIV/AIDS.

GABA (gamma-amino butyric acid) is an inhibitory neurotransmitter. This could account for *Sutherlandia*'s success in treating anxiety, stress, and depression, and for observed improvements in mood and well-being experienced by patients taking preparations from the plant.

SU1 is a novel triterpenoid isolated by members of the PhytoNova team that is showing promising biological activity.

A STUDY OF TOXICITY

To date, no severe adverse reaction to *Sutherlandia* in any form has ever been reported. Nevertheless, an independent safety study was conducted by South Africa's Medical Research Council because of the significant ethnobotanical background and availability of the plant, as well as the severity of the HIV/AIDS problem in the region. The study tested the effect of *Sutherlandia* on sixteen vervet monkeys in four groups, including one control. The monkeys were fed with dried *Sutherlandia* leaf powder for three months and exhibited no single indication of toxicity, even in the group fed nine times the dosage prescribed for the treatment of AIDS in humans. A massive dose of 500mg/kg by mouth was administered without any adverse effect. This is the first South African medicinal plant to be evaluated for toxicity using primates in a controlled study.[15]

The Indigenous Knowledge Systems (IKS) division of the Medical Research Council (MRC) of South Africa is committed to the scientific and clinical validation of promising indigenous medicinal plants. *Sutherlandia* is considered by IKS to have a long history of medicinal use going back at least 105 years. IKS acknowledges that a tonic made from the plants may be of value to people living with HIV/AIDS in terms of enhanced well-being, increased appetite and body mass, and increased tolerance for exercise. Use of *Sutherlandia* is contraindicated in pregnancy.[16]

The IKS was formed in 2001 and has collaborated successfully with traditional healers across the regions of Africa. So far it has identified twenty traditional healers across the region from the 300,000 that are estimated to be practicing on the continent. The select healers are encouraged to keep records of their consultations, and it is hoped they will train other healers to do so. A medicinal garden project has also been started where plants can be cultivated and identified. A library and computer systems are also being developed alongside a TM database called TRAMED III, which incorporates medicinal plant monographs.

Sutherlandia is not without its critics. Stuart Thomson, a holistic health researcher and director of the Gaia Research Institute in South Africa, has attacked the plant, the MRC trials, and PhytoNova. He says *Sutherlandia* is a "poison panacea" and that PhytoNova is unlawfully distributing a substance he believes is potentially toxic, as well as using people as guinea pigs. Thomson considers the MRC study to be invalid because the monkeys were not infected with HIV/AIDS and were studied for less than six months.[17] He also raises some questions on the safety of L-canavanine (see the box). But *Sutherlandia* taken under allopathic or traditional medical guidance would certainly seem to offer an alternative to sludgy liquids made of industrial solvents that sell like hotcakes on the streets of Johannesburg, peddled by those looking to exploit the numbers of desperate people living with HIV/AIDS.[18]

Of course, there are plants among Africa's flora and fauna that are toxic; efforts are being made to study and document these to avoid incorrect TM treatment of HIV/AIDS or indeed any illness. One such plant recorded to have toxic properties is *Callilepis laurealo* or *impila*.

FURTHER STUDIES

The novel triterpenoid SU1 (see box) isolated from *Sutherlandia* by the PhytoNova team has undergone three recent scientific studies.

- **Anticancer**. The University of British Columbia, Canada, has demonstrated that SU1 has anticancer activity.[19] This affirms *Sutherlandia*'s role as a helpful tonic that can be prescribed by healthcare professionals to patients with life-threatening diseases.
- **Antistress**. Researchers concluded that SU1 is an effective adaptogen (tonic that strengthens the body) capable of maintaining the body's stress hormones at a level where it functions optimally. The results provide scientific evidence of *Sutherlandia*'s stress-relieving properties and support the validity of indigenous knowledge.[20]
- **Antioxidant**. Pharmacologists found SU1 to be a powerful antioxidant with the potential to treat diseases that overproduce oxidants, such as autoimmune and infectious diseases.[21]

One *Sutherlandia* plant can treat ten people. Credo Mutwa of Phyto Nova says cultivating *Sutherlandia* is a question of sanding each little seed with fine sandpaper, then planting them, watering them, and letting them grow. He refuses to see his country destroyed by HIV and AIDS when nobody really knows the origins of the disease. He reminds critics that the bark of the *Cinchona* tree forms the natural chemical basis of quinine, which, when used correctly, is a successful treatment of malaria for many.[22] Since resistance to quinine has become more prevalent, the shrub *Artemesia* was discovered to contain an alkaloid, called artemesian, with even greater efficacy for the treatment of mefloquinine-resistant strains of malaria.

The MRC also plans a pilot clinical trial on the medicinal effects of *Sutherlandia* involving fifty people.[23] This was scheduled to begin in February 2002, pending a decision by the Governments Medical Approval Council. "A trial like this could act as a valuable template for other trials," the director of IKS, Dr. Matlalepula Matsabisa, told *New Scientist*. "The fact is people are already using it and will continue to whether or not the government approves trials."[24]

It appears that South Africa's first-line treatment of HIV/AIDS is *Sutherlandia*, which is local to the regions where it is needed most, and whose history as a beneficial traditional medicine puts it firmly in the hands of the people.

Hypericum Versus HIV/AIDS

AN ANCIENT WEED HAS DRAMATIC EFFECTS
ON VIRUSES WITH A LIPID ENVELOPE.

HYPERICUM EXTRACTS ARE ANTIRETROVIRAL

St. John's wort (*Hypericum perforatum*) is a yellow-flowered, five-petaled perennial that grows in Europe, Asia, and the United States; its star-shaped flowers bloom around the summer solstice. *Wort* is an old Anglo-Saxon name meaning herbal medicine. St. John's wort has gained a reputation as a reliable traditional treatment for mild depression due to an impressive cache of organic compounds. The small red dots on the flowers contain hypericin, which belongs to a group of compounds called napthodianthrones. Hypericin is an efficacious antiretroviral against a variety of viruses.[1]

A team of scientists from New York University Medical School and the Weizmann Institute in Israel studied the effect of hypericin and pseudohypericin extracted from St. John's wort on reverse transcriptase in mice. Both proved highly effective in preventing viral-induced diseases that follow infection of various retroviruses *in vivo* and *in vitro*.[2]

But unlike conventional reverse transcriptase therapies, hypericin and pseudohypericin have no effect against the transcription, translation, or transport of viral proteins to the cell membranes, and no effect on the polymerase (a vital DNA enzyme). What the compounds are most likely to do is interfere with the viral infection by deactivating the virus and preventing it from shedding, budding, or assembling at the cell membrane.

The scientists observed low toxicity *in vitro* and *in vivo* at concentrations "sufficient to produce dramatic antiviral effects in murine [mouse] tissue." The mice were given single injections of small doses of hypericin, which totally prevented the onset of Friend leukemia virus and radiation leukemia virus. After being infected with the viruses, the treated mice survived more than 240 days, compared to 15 to 30 days for untreated controls. Preliminary *in vitro* studies with pseudohypericin indicate that it can reduce the spread of HIV.[3]

Both hypericin and pseudohypericin interfere with one or more stages of viral infection by causing photochemical alterations of the capsid (protein coat of a virus particle), which inhibits the release of reverse transcriptase and prevents the reverse transcription of the genome within the target cell. Together, the napthodianthrones hypericin and pseudohypericin are called total hypericin (TH) and are responsible for the reddish color of all *Hypericum* extracts.

A trial was carried out on eighteen HIV-positive patients treated intravenously with 2ml of hypericin infusion twice a week, interspersed with oral doses of two tablets containing hypericin three times a day. Sixteen of the eighteen patients had stabilized or elevated CD4 and CD8 T-cell counts over the forty-month duration of the study. Only two people in the positive-response group experienced any opportunistic infection during the trial.[4] No viral complications such as herpes, cytomegalovirus, or Epstein-Barr virus were reported, and no cases of photosensitivity, neurological symptoms, or toxoplasmosis occurred.

ALTERNATIVE TREATMENT FOR THE SYMPTOMS OF HIV/AIDS

The dramatic effects of St. John's wort were documented by John James, the editor of *AIDS Treatment News*, who in 1989 tracked down all the existing data on HIV-positive individuals who were using or had used St. John's wort as an alternative medicinal treatment. He found nineteen people who had, with the help of their doctors, included or used the plant as partial or entire treatment for the symptoms of HIV/AIDS. Anecdotal evidence about the use of St. John's wort can be found on James's Web site (www.aids.org/atn/a-077-02.html). Here is one remarkable story he uncovered.

Of the nineteen people James found, four were in the care of Dr. David Payne, an osteopathic physician based in Arizona. The protocol for his AIDS patients was a standardized extract called Hyperforat, which was sold over the counter in Germany as an antidepressant. The recommended dose for depression is 20 to 30 drops three times a day, but under the guidance of the New York University researchers (above), Dr. Payne increased the dose for his HIV/AIDS patients to 40 drops three times a day, 120 drops per day total.

One of his patients, "Ted," was bedridden and being fed through a catheter. Ted was brought into Dr. Payne's office in a wheelchair and was very sick; he could not keep anything in his stomach and was wasting away. He was extremely fatigued, had no strength in his legs, and was suffering from mild neuropathy. Dr. Payne began hypericin treatment immediately, and within two weeks Ted walked into Dr. Payne's office and reported receiving only 30 percent of his nutrition via catheter. After two more weeks on the hypericin, he was able to drive himself the two-and-a-half-hour trip to his wife's workplace, eat a full diet, and do a little hiking as exercise. Hypericin was the only treatment that Ted received, as he could not tolerate AZT or dextran sulfate.

In 1990 an uncontrolled study assessed twenty-six HIV patients self-administering an over-the-counter *Hypericum* extract at a dose of 1mg per day TH equivalent.[5] At the end of four months, p24 antigenemia in two of the six initially positive patients disappeared. Both these patients had also been using AZT. Ten patients who had never taken AZT increased their mean CD4 cell count by 13 percent after one month and maintained this increase for the duration of the trial. For the remainder who used both AZT and TH, CD4 cell count fell significantly after a mild rise. One side effect was an elevation in liver enzyme counts in five patients, which returned to normal after one month without hypericin.

ACTION AGAINST COATED VIRUSES

The antiviral activity of hypericin is enhanced by the presence of light.[6] Three viruses were tested: murine cytomegalovirus, Sindbis virus, and HIV type 1. All were susceptible to hypericin, but antiviral activity *in vitro* was considerably enhanced in a dose-dependent manner by exposure to light. TH appears to inactivate the viral function via the generation of singlet oxygen upon illumination.[7] The antiviral activity of hypericin is directed at both the virions (fully assembled viruses) and virus-infected cells.[8]

155

The ring structure of hypericin, comprising quinone and phenolic groups (plant compounds), is necessary for the antiviral activity.[9]

It is thought that TH acts against viruses by impairing the assembly of intact viruses.[10] Furthermore, TH interferes with the processing of *gag*-encoded precursor polyproteins needed for viruses to reach the final stage of maturation.

Hypericin inhibits only viruses that have a lipid envelope—for example, herpes simplex viruses 1 and 2, cytomegalovirus, influenza A virus, hepatitis B, chicken pox, shingles (herpes zoster), and Epstein-Barr virus, as well as HIV-1. Viruses without this protein envelope or naked viruses are unaffected by hypericin.[11] Although not fully understood, the antiviral properties of TH are thought to be due to the inhibition of an enzyme called protease kinase C during the viral infection of cells.[12]

Hypericum extracts can inhibit viruses in other ways: hypericin inhibits the signaling pathway that has an immunosuppressive effect on the host immune system.[13] The combination of the photodynamic and lipohilic (belonging to napthodianthrones) hypericin binding with cell membranes results in a loss of viral infectivity and an inability to retrieve the reverse transcriptase action from the virion.[14]

A study of twenty-four HIV patients in Thailand determined the maximum tolerated dose of TH. This was found to be 0.05mg/kg body weight.[15] But mild photosensitivity of short duration on exposure to sunlight was observed in three-quarters of the patients. The dose was then raised to 0.16mg/kg, which produced intolerable symptoms of photosensitivity in two patients and mild symptoms in the remainder.

PHOTOTOXICITY

Hypericin is recognized as a phototoxic substance that can cause photosensitization, especially in fair-skinned people. People exposed to the sun may burn or tan faster after oral consumption of *Hypericum*. A study found that 600mg three times a day reduced tanning time by 21 percent.[16] In a study of 3,250 patients, only 2.4 percent reported allergic reaction, tiredness, gastrointestinal irritation, or restlessness.[17]

Studies using synthetic hypericin have not been encouraging.[18] Phototoxicity varying in severity developed in all participants. A consistent change in viral endpoints with injection or oral dosing of synthetic hypericin was not observed.

AN EFFECTIVE, NONTOXIC ANTIDEPRESSANT

Hypericum has long been used as an antidepressant. It inhibits a neuro-transmitter called monoamine oxidase and catechol methyltransferase (COMT), which lowers the stress hormone cortisol and affects GABA receptors in the brain. A study compared 600mg of a standardized *Hypericum* extract twice daily with 50mg of imipramine, a conventional antidepressant; both were able to improve depression. A measurement of anxiety and physical symptoms relating to anxiety showed that *Hypericum* was better tolerated, with 34.6 percent of those on *Hypericum* reporting adverse events, compared with 81.4 percent of those on imipramine.[19]

Hypericum has very low toxicity. Animals given 2g/kg per day of dried *Hypericum* for up to a year showed no indication of toxic effects.[20] Doses of 3g/kg or more of ground dried *Hypericum* caused photosensitivity in four- to six-month-old calves.[21]

There have been no reliable reports of hypericism (severe dermatitis in domestic animals attributable to photosensitivity from eating St. John's wort) in humans taking oral doses of *Hypericum*. A therapeutic dose of *Hypericum* is approximately thirty to fifty times smaller than the dose needed to induce phototoxicity in calves.[22]

Hypericum has received mixed reviews as an alternative medicine, but sales increased tenfold in two years, from $20 million in 1995 to $200 million in 1997. Perhaps it is time that the ancient *Hypericum*, brought to our attention by Hippocrates, the "father of medicine," and its multifaceted store of compounds—catechin, epicatechin, beta-sitosteral, TH, isohypericin, and protohypericin; the flavonoids hyperforin, quercetin, rutin, and biflavones; monoterpenes, GABA, B_2, melatonin, and essential oils—received a percentage of the billions of dollars spent on AIDS research to investigate just how its antiretroviral properties work and how it can be used effectively either alone or in combination with conventional medicine to ease the symptoms of HIV/AIDS.

St. John's wort is contraindicated for use with the following medicines: cyclosporin, warfarin, oral contraceptives, theophylline, digoxin, and indinavir. It should also not be used with the protease inhibitors ritonavir, nelinavir, and saquinavir, or the non-nucleosides nevirapine and efavirenz. Interactions are also possible with antidepressants, migraine treatments, and the anticonvulsants phenobarbitone, phenytoin, and carbamazepine. The U.K. Medicines Control Agency has issued guidelines for doctors and for HIV patients that patients receiving both conventional medicine and taking any form of *Hypericum* must have a viral-load test to assess the effects of the herbal medicine. Also, those taking *Hypericum* long term need periodic tests of liver function.

Therapeutic Mushrooms

POWERFUL EXTRACTS FROM FUNGI ARE BRIDGING THE
GAP BETWEEN TRADITIONAL AND CONVENTIONAL
TREATMENTS OF CANCER AND HIV/AIDS.

IMMUNE POTENTIATORS

It has become increasingly apparent that various immune disorders, including cancers and AIDS, are not effectively treated by the use of cytocidal (cell-killing) chemotherapeutics or immunological agents alone. According to Professor Goro Chihara of Teikyo University in Japan, augmentation of the immune system comes about through substances that enhance the body's defense mechanisms, which he terms host defense potentiators (HDPs). Cytokines such as interleukin-2 (IL-2) or tumor necrosis factor are not categorized as HDPs, as their action is generally localized and not particularly selective (see the chapter "Vaccinating People Against Their Own Genes").[1]

Chihara isolated and purified a primary polysaccharide called lentinan from the edible mushroom *Letinus edodes* (shiitake) in the late 1960s. Lentinan is considered to be an HDP, but it is thought to be too toxic for long-term clinical use. In 1971, a search for a less toxic HDP turned up the active principle from the mushroom *Coriolus versicolor*, which was extracted and named polysaccharide krestin (PSK). PSK comprises high-molecular-weight protein-bound polysaccharides known as beta-glucans that can enhance immunity and help slow the spread of cancer cells.[2]

C. *versicolor* (*kawaratake*) is an ancient Asian herbal remedy that has a reputation for anticancer properties, perhaps as powerful as some chemotherapy treatments. It is antimicrobial and antiviral, and is an antioxidant that blocks the action of free radicals (activated oxygen molecules in the cells). The fruiting body of the mushroom contains the PSK, which is formed by numerous long-chain sugar molecules that appear to increase the number and activity of T-cells and natural killer (NK) cells. PSK gained commercial approval in Japan in the 1980s for treating various cancers and for use in conjunction with surgery, chemotherapy, and radiation therapy.[3]

CORIOLUS SUPPORTS NK CELLS

There is little on C. *versicolor* in peer-reviewed journals, but studies on PSK have been reported. At the University of Texas Center for Alternative Medicine Research in Cancer, a review of eight randomized trials found that patients who received PSK with conventional treatments survived longer and enjoyed longer disease-free periods.[4]

Two studies in Japan on colorectal and gastric cancers compared PSK to placebo. The first found that patients with colorectal cancer who received PSK survived longer.[5] The second involved forty-two hospitals and 260 patients who had stomach-cancer surgery. Those who received PSK with chemotherapy had higher five-year disease-free and survival rates than those receiving chemotherapy alone.[6]

Dr. Jean Munro, the founder of Breakspear Hospital in the United Kingdom, is a leading specialist in chronic fatigue and immune dysfunction syndrome (CFIDS) and has observed the low levels of NK cells in her patients. From May to September 2000, she treated fifteen CFIDS-diagnosed patients with six 500mg tablets per day of *Coriolus* supplement (three tablets morning and evening, totaling 3g per day) for fifteen days. This was followed for a further forty-five days by a decrease to three tablets per day. The patients were then assessed according to changes in their NK-cell activity, measured in lytic units.[7]

In healthy individuals, NK levels are 41 ± 19 units, whereas cancer patients have levels of 5 ± 6 units, and CFIDS patients have levels of

13 ± 6 units. After treatment with *Coriolus* supplement, the average NK-cell activity of the fifteen CFIDS patients was 31 units, a significant rise toward healthy levels. It appears that *Coriolus* affects the TH1 immune response's ability to transform CD8 suppressor cells into NK cells[8] and is able to relieve the fatigue symptoms of CFIDS patients. *Coriolus* supplement is also being studied in lung-cancer patients undergoing radiotherapy and patients with chronic fatigue syndrome.

Coriolus supplement has been used in clinical studies on long-term HIV-positive survivors since 1999.[9] Physiologist and acupuncturist Majilke Pfeiffer founded the Centrum voor Gereeskunde in Amsterdam to bridge the gap between complementary and conventional medicine in the treatment of immune-deficiency disorders. Her protocol for treating HIV-positive patients is three tablets of *Coriolus* supplement twice a day for two weeks and then three tablets once a day in the morning for a minimum of twelve months. Patients also receive acupuncture treatments once a month. All patients have CD4 levels and viral load measured four times a year. The results from a study started in January 2000 are encouraging (see Table 4).

In a typical case study, a forty-one-year-old man had been HIV-positive for three years; his main health problems were candidiasis and diarrhea. After six months of taking *Coriolus* supplement, acupuncture, and Chinese herbs, his viral load was down from 152,000 to 31,000, and his fatigue, candidiasis, and diarrhea had resolved. After one year, his symptoms had not returned; he was well and started some sports. He is continuing with traditional Chinese medicine (TCM) treatment.

All the patients except two received TCM comprising *Coriolus* supplement, Chinese herbs, and acupuncture as sole treatments. The two who received both TCM and conventional drugs came off highly active antiretroviral therapy (HAART) due to side effects. All patients had common symptoms of candidiasis and diarrhea that improved with the TCM protocol. One patient also suffered from herpes zoster and one had hepatitis C; both conditions improved significantly with TCM.

Pfeiffer explains that supporting the immune system of the patient with TCM rather than attacking the cause of the disease is helping her patients. She says that the intestinal flora also plays an important role in resistance to disease, which has often been damaged by past use of

Table 4. Long-Term HIV-Positive Patient Response to a TCM Protocol Using *Coriolus* Supplement

Patient	A	B	C	D*	E	F	G**
Years HIV+	3	5	17	11	13	17	16
CD4 count							
Jan	460	650	600	600	450	—	60
May	540	700	680	320	520	450	20
Aug	520	650	700	550	560	540	100
Dec	630	680	720	480	630	590	80
Viral load							
Jan	31,000	1,100	10,000	10,000	12,000	—	125,000
May	22,000	800	6,500	15,000	10,000	22,000	92,000
Aug	12,000	2,400	5,000	90,000	10,000	15,000	20,000
Dec	3,200	0	2,400	42,000	6,200	8,300	12,000

* This female patient, thirty-two years old, received HAART medication from January 1998 to December 1999 because her CD4 count had dropped from 700 to 300 and she had high viral load. With HAART medication, her CD4 count rose to 850 and her viral load fell to 50. She ceased HAART because of increasing side effects, notably lipodystrophy and neuropathy. With *Coriolus* treatment, she was able to resume work and visit the gym three times a week. Her lipodystrophy improved slowly and her neuropathy disappeared.

** This male patient had tried every available conventional medicine to treat HIV over the past twelve years. While he was taking HAART, his viral load was 125,000 and CD4 count 60. He suffered from multiple opportunistic infections and all the side effects associated with conventional AIDS drugs. By September his CD4 count had increased to 100, and his viral load had decreased from 300,000 to 92,0000. His weight increased from 88 to 92.5 pounds (40 to 42kg), and he could walk every day for up to forty-five minutes.

antibiotics. She frequently recommends supplements that assist the recovery of intestinal flora, including probiotics (see "Eating Well for Health" and "Probiotics for Life After HIV/AIDS").

MAITAKE SYNERGISTIC WITH CHEMOTHERAPY

The maitake mushroom (*Grifola frondosa*) has fruiting bodies that overlap each other and look like butterflies in a wild dance; maitake means "dancing mushroom." Like *Coriolus*, the maitake mushroom is known for its immunostimulating effects. It contains the powerful immune activators alpha and beta D-glucans, with beta D-glucans predominating. The complex polysaccharides in the maitake have a unique structure and have been studied in cancer prevention and as an adjunct to diabetes treatment.[10] Powdered maitake has been shown to enhance the activity of T-cells by 1.4, 1.86, and 1.6 times in different studies, as well as NK cells and macrophages. It is also used in Japan to support patients undergoing chemotherapy and has the potential to reduce pain and nausea, extend life, regress tumor growth, and work synergistically with conventional treatments.[11]

SHIITAKE AGAINST VIRUSES

The beta D-glucans from *Lentinus edodes* (shiitake) were used in a phase I/II trial of HIV-positive patients at San Francisco General Hospital. The ninety patients in the trial, all of whom had CD4 levels between 200 and 500, were between the ages of eighteen and sixty and were suffering from opportunistic infections. Side effects of *Lentinus* treatment were mainly mild, but with ten-minute-long infusions, there were nine side effects severe enough to be reported to the FDA. Infusions carried out over a thirty-minute period, however, caused no side effects. Four patients dropped out of the study by choice, and all adverse effects were relieved after medication had been discontinued for twenty-four hours. Patients showed a trend toward increases in CD4 cells, and some patients showed neutrophil activity. In view of the positive effect on certain markers and the lack of adverse events such as anemia, pancreatitis, or neuropathy, the authors recommended a long-term clinical study of lentinan in combination with didanosine or AZT in HIV-positive patients.[12]

A study was carried out on 107 people with CD4 counts between 200 and 500 who received the anti-HIV drug didanosine (400mg/day) with the addition at week six of lentinan (2mg IV per week) for between twenty-four and eighty weeks. The control group received didanosine only. The controls experienced CD4 count increases that remained significant to week sixteen, while in the combination group, CD4 count increases remained significant to week thirty-eight.[13]

An extract of the culture medium of *Lentinus edodes* mycelia significantly blocked the release of infectious HSV-1 in African green monkey kidney cells. It is thought that the expression of glycoproteins B, E, and I (viral proteins) were blocked at a late stage in the virus replication cycle in treated cells.[14]

OTHER MUSHROOMS

Other therapeutic mushrooms containing high-molecular-weight protein-bound polysaccharides that are powerful adaptogens are *Cordyceps sinesis* (tochukas), indigenous to Nepal, and *Ganoderma lucidium* (reishi). Extract of reishi in a hot-water solution contains 50 percent polysac-charides that stimulate the immune system. In a study of 355 hepatitis patients receiving reishi extracts, 92 percent showed an improvement. Reishi is also terpene-rich and is a useful treatment for hypertension, bronchitis, bronchial asthma, and allergies.

Philip Calder, professor of nutritional immunology at Southampton University in England, appears to have coined the term *immunonutrition*. Immunonutrition refers to the potential to modulate the activity of the immune system by interventions with specific nutrients, which is indeed gaining in popularity[15] (see "Eating Well for Health").

"MUSHROOM" TEA

Kombucha is not really a mushroom but a multispecies community of yeasts and bacteria living in an extracellular matrix. It is known for its healing properties and is commonly referred to as "tea of immortality" (China, 221 BCE). Its widespread use in Russia among the peasants led to reports of no cancer in their communities.[16] Kombucha can be pro-duced and used freely as a home remedy, which may explain why very little scientific interest has been expressed in its rich content of enzymes, folic acid, gluconic acid, glucuronic acid, lactic acid, amino acids, vitamins B_1, B_2, B_3, B_6, and B_{12}, and vitamin C.

For therapeutic purposes, the whole fruit of the mushroom is used either in a capsule or in tea; intake ranges from 1,000 to 9,000mg per day. The FDA has rejected many mycological products in tea, powder, or tablet form from China and Japan because standardization, industrial toxins, and pesticides in the raw materials are an issue.

AIDS Therapy from Cheap Generics

CONVENTIONAL COMBINATION TREATMENTS FOR HIV/AIDS
COST $22 000 PER PATIENT PER YEAR IN THE US.
DO CHEAPER AND LESS TOXIC DRUGS EXIST?

NEW USES FOR CHEAP OLD DRUGS

A quintet of older drugs could make a cheap and safe alternative to current anti-HIV drug cocktails, claim Dr. Aldar Bourinbaiar and Dr. Vichai Jirathitikal of Immunitor Corporation in Thailand, which created the V1 AIDS vaccine (see "The 'Pink Panacea': An AIDS Vaccine?").

In a paper published in *Current Pharmaceutical Design* in 2003, the two scientists reviewed evidence suggesting that these old, widely available conventional drugs might have antiretroviral and immune modulating properties, which could help recover the immune system of HIV/AIDS patients.[1]

WARFARIN

Warfarin is a synthetic drug derived from the naturally occurring coumarins found in a wide variety of plant species worldwide. Coumarins are the parent organic compounds that work as natural pesticides in plants such as lavender, grasses like sweet clover, and food plants like strawberries and lemons. In 1868, coumarins were synthesised in the laboratory to make perfumes and flavoring. When combined with glucose,

165

they produce glycosides, which are anticancer, antifungus, and anti-coagulant. All structurally related coumarins show potent anti-HIV activity. The use of coumarins as an immune support accompanying standard chemotherapy treatment has significantly improved survival rates of colon-cancer patients. More recently, warfarin has been used as an anticoagulating drug in the treatment of heart disease and stroke.

There is some anecdotal evidence suggesting that a small daily dose of 2mg of warfarin does not affect prothrombin time, a lab test to monitor blood coagulation in HIV patients, but does significantly lower viral loads.

Warfarin possesses four essential properties for fighting HIV: inhibition of serine protease, aspartyl protease, reverse transcriptase, and integrase, all of which are central to the virus's ability to replicate.

An average protease inhibitor used in triple-drug treatments of HIV costs between $10 and $20 per day, in contrast to a daily dose of 2mg warfarin, which costs as little as 10 cents.

Reverse transcriptase (RT) inhibitors are also essential in the successful treatment of HIV/AIDS. By far the most prescribed RT inhibitor is AZT, which has side effects in up 75 percent of patients with HIV/AIDS.

Warfarin is of further value in the treatment of cognitive functions in HIV/AIDS patients. A daily dose of warfarin appears to improve the fluency of speech and mental aptitude of patients suffering from progressive dementia associated with full-blown AIDS disease.

Bourinbaiar and Jirathitikal found that a combination of warfarin with compounds whose anti-HIV effects they had discovered, such as cimetidine and levamisole, seem to enhance the beneficial immune effect.

CIMETIDINE

Cimetidine (Tagamet) is an over-the-counter antacid or antiulcer drug, and as such inhibits gastric acid secretion via histamine-type (H2) receptors on parietal cells (in the stomach). Cimetidine was developed as part of a research effort led by Nobel laureate Sir James Black and was the first H2-antagonist to receive approval from the Food and Drug Administration in 1977. Because of its excellent safety record, it is now widely available as an over-the-counter drug.

Cimetidine first came to the attention of Bourinbaiar and Jirathitikal when they observed the inhibition of human T-cell leukemia virus (HTLV-1) secretion from chronically infected cells. This led them to the idea that viral release is regulated in the same way as gastric acid secretion, and to discover that cimetidine has broad antiretroviral activity.

Further studies revealed that cimetidine, unlike AZT, which was used as a control, produced no cytotoxicity even at the highest dose tested (1mM). According to the researchers, this is an exceptional drug index that cannot be matched by any drugs currently used in the treatment of HIV/AIDS. Twice-daily doses of 200mg of cimetidine provide steady IC50 levels (concentration producing 50 percent inhibition) for HIV replication.

It appears that the success of H2 antagonists tested for antiviral activity depends on the imidazole nucleus. Some, although not all, non-nucleoside reverse transcriptase inhibitors (NNRTIs) possess the special chemical structures, called imidazole rings, that are present in cimetidine. It is thus likely that cimetidine acts like an NNRTI and has the ability to treat HIV infection.

NNRTIs have a reputation for rapidly eliciting resistance due to mutations of the amino acids surrounding the NNRTIs' binding site. So emerging strains of resistant HIV can be confronted if the NNRTIs are combined with other anti-HIV agents such as cimetidine.

The combination of warfarin and cimetidine was previously thought to be incompatible, but there have been no reports of adverse reactions at low doses of cimetidine and 2mg of warfarin in more than 100 available references in the TOXLINE database. In fact, cimetidine has caused anemia in only 2.3 per 100,000 people, as opposed to 70 percent of HIV patients treated with AZT.[2] In trials, cimetidine significantly enhanced a variety of immune functions both *in vivo* and *in vitro* and was successful in partially restoring the immune function in thirty-three AIDS patients.[3] Cimetidine sells over the counter for 20 cents per 400mg pill; in China, the pills may be purchased in bulk for as little as $18 per kilogram.

LEVAMISOLE

Levamisole was synthesized in the early 1960s and was used primarily for the treatment of intestinal worms in animals. In the 1990s, levamisole was approved for human medicinal use to provide immune support for colon-cancer patients. Bourinbaiar and colleagues, aware that it contained the same imidazole ring as cimetidine, surmised that it might also have anti-HIV activity. They found the IC50 of levamisole to be around 0.1 µM, and there was no toxicity at the highest dose of 1 µM. The drug was effective against several lab strains and primary isolates of HIV-1.[4]

Chronic daily doses of levamisole, however, appeared to have an accumulated toxic effect, usually severe nausea and granulocytopenia (a reduction of granulocytes, a kind of white blood cells). In general, low once-weekly doses of the drug are well tolerated.

Interestingly, levamisole can either enhance or suppress the immune system depending on the administered dose. Many studies have found beneficial effects of levamisole in various immune deficiency disorders. Similarly, the drug used alone, or in combination with interferon and other anti-inflammatory drugs, significantly improves the healing of eye and skin lesions caused by herpes simplex and zoster virus. Levamisole is also strikingly effective against autoimmune diseases such as rheumatoid arthritis and systemic lupus erythematosus.

Other studies, however, have found no benefit from levamisole.

Since 1985, levamisole has undergone sporadic tests with AIDS patients with conflicting results. Some trials report no effect, while others have found beneficial effects.

Bourinbaiar and Jirathitikal conclude that levamisole may have both immune-modulating and antiviral activities. But caution must be exercised in using this drug, they say, because "the dosage, administration schedule, gender, and many other variables seem to have a serious influence on the outcome of the therapy."[5]

For human use, levamisole costs $6 per pill, but the same pill for animal use costs just 6 cents. So the cost for treating a sheep for one year is $1, but treating a human for one year would cost $1,200.

ACETAMINOPHEN

Acetaminophen was first synthesized in 1878 as an intermediary compound in the manufacture of synthetic aniline dyes. Its analgesic or painkilling property was identified some fifteen years later, but its clinical application was not established until 1949, when a study by Nobel laureates William Brodie and Julius Axelrod was published. In the 1960s, it was made available as an over-the-counter drug. Brand names for acetaminophen include Paracetamol, Panadol, and Tylenol. It is a nontoxic, broad-spectrum pain reliever with few or no side effects at therapeutic doses. It is thought to cause fewer side effects than aspirin, a common nonsteroidal anti-inflammatory (NSAID) drug.

It is not fully understood how acetaminophen works, but it is believed to inhibit prostaglandin synthesis or the actions of chemical mediators or other substances that sensitize the pain receptors to mechanical or chemical stimulation. In the course of a study to identify a serine protease for use in contraceptive creams, Bourinbaiar and Jirathitikal discovered that acetaminophen, which was being used as a negative control, displayed significant anti-HIV activity. The antiviral effect was specific, and almost 100 percent inhibition was observed at 1mM (150 µg/ml), while IC50 was 20 µg/ml, which is satisfied by the standard dosage of a 650mg pill every six hours.[6]

Studies of acetaminophen have shown it to be nontoxic even in the highest dose of 1mM tested, and it has been used to counteract toxicity in AIDS patients treated with AZT. No further toxicity occurred in the patients, but the anti-HIV activity of acetaminophen was not studied in these cases.[7]

It is not yet clear how acetaminophen affects HIV replication, but it is thought to behave in a similar way to RT inhibitors that inhibit the synthesis of DNA from RNA.

As far as cost is concerned, these familiar painkillers may well turn out to be the cheapest of all currently available anti-RT drugs.

GRAMICIDIN

Gramicidin D was the first clinically identified antibiotic, predating penicillin by one year. It was isolated from the soil bacterium *Bacillis brevis* by Rene Dubois (hence the *D*), in 1939. Gramicidins are short peptides of fifteen alternating L- and D-amino acids that are synthesized outside the genetic coding route for all other peptides and polypeptides in living organisms. The D-amino acids are unnatural in that they do not occur in proteins encoded in the genome of organisms. There are several kinds of gramicidins, differing in amino acid sequence. They usually exist as molecular complexes of two peptides. These linear gramicidins are related to the cyclic (ring-shaped) gramicidin S discovered later in the former Soviet Union.

Gramicidin acts by causing potassium to flow out from the target cell, thus killing it. Because of its unique construction, it has never been implicated in the emergence of resistant bacteria, like so many newer antibiotics.

It was first used in the United States for the treatment of gram-positive infections and was also widely used in over-the-counter throat lozenges, dentifrices, and mouthwashes. Today it is available by prescription only as a treatment for skin and eye infections. In Russia, gramicidin S is available over the counter as a spermicide, which can be used in combination with condoms and diaphragms. It can be applied topically as an antimicrobial to treat skin infections caused by viral or fungal sexually transmitted diseases and also burns.

Gramicidin has been in clinical use for over sixty years; it is nontoxic when administered topically or orally. Some medical opinions, however, suggest toxicity with systemic use. This may have been because gramicidin was used in combination with other drugs, which caused side effects. More recent studies have shown that systemic doses of gramicidin are well tolerated and effective in the treatment of experimental malaria in mice; gramicidin injections cleared the malaria parasite in four days.[8,9] It is hoped that gramicidin can be a potent treatment for both AIDS and malaria, particularly in Africa, where both diseases are endemic.

Due to the presence of unnatural D-amino acids, gramicidin has a remarkable resistance to peptide-cleaving proteases found in the body, such as blood, pus, urine, and saliva. It has a broad pH range (acid to alkaline) and remains active for ten years at room temperature.

Bourinbaiar and his co-workers have shown that gramicidin is highly effective against HIV and herpes simplex viruses at nontoxic nanogram doses. The IC50 of gramicidin against three herpes simplex isolates was 0.3 µg/ml. At an even lower dose of 10 µg/ml, it was active against both lab strains of HIV and clinical isolates. When gramicidin was compared with the most popular anti-HIV spermicide, N9, it was found to be 1,000 times more effective.[10–12] N9 could display antiviral activity only in doses that were toxic to cells. Despite N9's equivalence to household bleach, a toxic substance not normally topically applied to skin, it continues to be evaluated as a spermicide in clinical trials.

Thus, gramicidin may be a safe and more efficient microbicide and spermicide than N9. Its use as a vaginal suppository would make an extremely cheap and efficient prophylactic or "barrier method" against HIV and other STDs. A supply of 3kg would be sufficient for one year's use, and the cost is negligible. Gramicidin D already has U.S. FDA approval for topical use, and cyclic gramicidin S has been used in Russia as a spermicidal preparation.

Gramicidin possesses a formidable list of attractive properties, all of which are relevant against emerging diseases. It is anti-STD, antifungal, antiprotozoan (malaria), and is poorly absorbed by the skin, reducing the risk of irritation. It enhances skin tissue healing and resists and inhibits proteolytic enzymes, which break down proteins in the body.

This sixty-year-old drug has now come of age, and its antiviral properties need to be confirmed in clinical trials.

Exercise Versus AIDS

Evidence is emerging on how exercise may help treat and prevent AIDS. If so, the simplest and most widely available and affordable natural "vaccine" is being ignored.

BEATING THE DEAD ENDS IN
AIDS THERAPY AND PREVENTION

The most effective way to control the HIV/AIDS pandemic would be the development of a safe and effective HIV vaccine. Unfortunately, despite enormous scientific and financial resources being deployed worldwide in the scientific establishment over the past fifteen years, no vaccine candidate is on the immediate horizon[1,2] (but see the chapter "The 'Pink Panacea': An AIDS Vaccine?"). There are also strong indications that the AIDS vaccines currently widely tested in humans are not only ineffective but also harmful[3–5] (see "The Dangers of AIDS Vaccine Trials," "AIDS Vaccines, or Slow Bioweapons?" "Controversy Breaks over AIDS Vaccine Trials," and "Vaccinating People Against Their Own Genes"). In addition, current medical therapy for HIV disease is extremely toxic, with multiple side effects and drug interactions (see "Anti-HIV Drugs Do More Harm Than Good"). Finally, it is very expensive and carries risks of developing drug-resistant HIV strains.

It is clearly desirable to pursue other inexpensive, less-toxic, nondrug approaches to slow the spread of HIV infection and to decrease the burden of HIV infection and treatment.

One solution may come from certain antibodies that appear to be directly involved in controlling HIV disease progression.[6,7] These antibodies have specific affinity, or cross-reactivity, to the HIV-1 envelope protein (gp120 surface antigen, residues 280–302, designated peptide NTM), but they may be naturally occurring autoantibodies (antibodies generated against the individual's own antigens) against a small protein molecule that acts to dilate the blood vessels in the intestine, the vasoactive intestinal peptide (VIP).[8,9]

It so happens that aerobic exercise training stimulates the formation of these anti-VIP/NTM antibodies in both normal (HIV-negative) and HIV-positive individuals, and perhaps both could benefit from such exercise.[10,11]

Increased levels of anti-VIP/NTM antibodies induced by exercise may have two beneficial effects. First, in HIV-negative individuals, the anti-VIP/NTM antibodies could bind HIV particles in circulation and prevent them from reaching their target cell, thereby reducing the risk of infection with HIV and decreasing transmission of the disease. Second, in HIV-positive individuals, increased levels of anti-VIP/NTM could slow HIV disease progression and reconstitute the damaged immune system.

Aerobic exercise may be an important, inexpensive, nontoxic, widely available frontline defense and therapy against HIV/AIDS. By acting as an immune stimulant (for both HIV-positive and HIV-negative individuals), it creates a type of "natural vaccine" that, if widely adopted, could contribute to a worldwide slowdown of the AIDS pandemic.

HIV AND AIDS DISEASE

The first step in HIV infection involves the gp120 on the outer envelope of the virus binding to receptors on the cell surface of the host, allowing HIV to enter the cell. The central portion of the gp120 molecule has an immunoglobulin-like structure, which facilitates participation in the immune network. Immediately after infection, HIV tries to produce a fit to the host idiotype (individual type) by producing thousands of variants of gp120. This process of adaptation usually takes years, and during this time, the host immune system is more or less able to control the HIV disease.

In some HIV-infected persons, this period is short, and in others it can be quite long, giving rise to the designations "slow" and "fast" disease progression (see "Surviving and Thriving with HIV"). After this latent period, a separate fraction of viruses will be established whose gp120 carries the host idiotype.[12–14] This population of HIV becomes accepted by the host immune system as "self" and is therefore protected from the host's immune attack. Even worse, these gp120 molecules are included in the regulation of the immune network, destabilizing its vital components and accelerating progression of disease.[15] In this way, HIV may escape from the latent period and progressively destroy the immune system of the infected person.

The gp120 protein represents the key component of all AIDS vaccine candidates that are currently in clinical trials. As the variants of gp120 are produced by the HIV infection, the vaccine antibodies may have the effect of disarming the immune system's antiviral response and thus increasing the likelihood of rapid disease progression.[16–18] This phenomenon has been seen in gp120 vaccine volunteers who later became infected with HIV[19,20] and would certainly reduce the utility of an HIV vaccine in AIDS prevention (see "The Dangers of AIDS Vaccine Trials").

USEFUL MOLECULAR MIMIC AND AUTOANTIBODIES IN HIV DISEASE

If an Achilles' heel exists in HIV, it might be in the central portion of gp120 (residues 280–302, designated as peptide NTM[21]). This portion of the molecule is highly conserved in all known HIV variants and appears to be crucial for viral infectivity. In fact, researchers have demonstrated that minimal changes in this sensitive peptide region completely abolish HIV infectivity. Unfortunately, this part of gp120 is not immunogenic in humans[22] because the immune system treats this part of gp120 as "self," possibly due to peptide NTM's similarity to several human proteins.[23] However, an antibody found in both HIV-positive and HIV-negative individuals seems to have reactivity to this region of the gp120 molecule.

A computer-assisted search of the Swiss-Prot database reveals VIP as the best match to NTM among currently analyzed human proteins.[24,25] The antibodies reacting to NTM may therefore be autoantibodies against VIP.

VIP is a small, naturally occurring peptide that plays several important roles in the human body, as a vasodilator (dilates blood vessels), a neurotransmitter, and a modulator of the immune system.

VIP stimulates natural killer (NK) cells in the immune system (among the first line of defense against infection) and also the production of cytokine, a hormone that influences the activity of cells in the immune system. VIP therefore plays a very important role in modulating the immune system.

The HIV protein gp120 is sufficiently similar to VIP to serve as a molecular mimic and interfere with its function. The main consequence of this mimicry is to undermine the NK cells, making them dysfunctional, which is common in HIV-infected subjects. Gp120 has been found to inhibit the ability of NK cells to kill infected cells, and this inhibition also affects the production of the proinflammatory cytokine IFN-γ,[26] which enlists the help of other cells in the immune system to fight the infection.

Thus, increase in circulating VIP can counteract the effects of the HIV gp120 by overcoming the latter's inhibition of NK cells and by stimulating the production of VIP autoantibodies, which can also bind gp120 and prevent it from binding to NK cells.

Finally, both VIP and the peptide NTM have been previously identified as possessing sequence characteristics responsible for the interaction between HIV and the CD4 receptor,[27] which represents the first step in the process of infection.

It has also been demonstrated that sera from HIV-negative asthma patients contains high levels of natural anti-VIP antibodies with peptide NTM reactivity. A recent study on sera from 393 HIV-negative blood donors found that approximately 5 percent (21 of 393) contained significant levels of the anti-VIP/NTM antibodies, corresponding to two standard deviations above average.

For HIV-positive individuals, anti-VIP/NTM antibodies appear to strongly correlate with progression of HIV disease, suggesting that the immune system is attempting to overcome the infection. HIV patients in the first stage of illness (characterized by CD4 lymphocyte count greater than 500/µl), when the immune system is efficiently controlling HIV, have very low levels of anti-VIP/NTM reactive antibodies, similar to levels in normal HIV-negative people.[28]

The level of these antibodies significantly increases in disease stages corresponding to CD4 values between 200 and 500/µl. Below that CD4 level (less than 200/µl), however, the amount of anti-VIP/NTM antibody sharply decreases. In the terminal stages of AIDS disease, NTM-reactive antibodies in sera of HIV-positive patients appear to be significantly decreased.

The spectrum of antibodies against HIV gp120 differs between those who remained healthy for at least ten years and those who developed AIDS within five years of infection;[29] antibodies recognizing the peptide 280–306 of HIV-1 gp120 (overlapping NTM) are significantly more prevalent in asymptomatic carriers than in AIDS patients. Thus, these antibodies may be a factor contributing to the delay of progression to AIDS disease.

EXERCISE AS A NATURAL SOURCE OF VIP/NTM-REACTIVE ANTIBODIES

A unique method to produce high titers of VIP/NTM-reactive antibodies may be available to both HIV-negative and HIV-positive individuals. In 1988, Paul and Said reported that autoantibodies to VIP were present in plasma from 29.6 percent of healthy (HIV-negative) human subjects who habitually performed aerobic muscular exercise, compared to 2.3 percent of healthy subjects who did not.[30] The exercise involved running, cycling, swimming, aerobic dancing, and/or weight training for three or more workouts per week for a year or more prior to the study. The antigenic stimulus for the formation of these autoantibodies could not be identified from these authors' data. Acute exercise, however, has been shown to be associated with a brisk increase in plasma levels of VIP.[31,32] It is therefore possible that the antibodies may have been produced in response to increased VIP levels during exercise.

EFFECT OF AEROBIC EXERCISE TRAINING ON HIV-POSITIVE INDIVIDUALS

Several studies on aerobic exercise training in HIV-positive individuals have demonstrated that it is safe and effective and has a number of beneficial outcomes.[33–47] The aerobic exercise fitness improvements include a 10 to 25 percent improvement in lactic acidosis threshold (a sign of fatigue) and a 5 to 10 percent increase in maximal oxygen uptake, depending on the exercise training intensity. In addition, despite concerns about the stress of aerobic exercise on already damaged immune systems (specifically, increases in infections, morbidity, or mortality), there have been no documented adverse effects of aerobic exercise training in HIV-positive patients at either moderate or heavy exercise training levels.[48] The available literature clearly supports the idea that aerobic exercise is well tolerated by HIV-positive individuals.

There are indications that exercise can stabilize CD4 cell count in HIV-infected individuals. Studies showed that people with CD4 cells between 200 and 500/µl seemed to benefit the most from an exercise program. A pilot study found that the mean change in CD4 percentage over a twenty-four-month interval for weight lifters was −3.1 percent compared with −5.9 percent for runners.[49] The same researchers also reported a case of a long-term survivor (twelve years HIV-positive), a triathlete with a rigorous daily exercise regimen who demonstrated very low viral burden as reflected in nondetectable HIV RNA quantitative PCR and increase in CD4 during six years from 3 to 50/µl.[50] There was also a report that exercise facilitated a return of the CD4 cell count to more normal levels.[51]

A large study involving 415 individuals (156 HIV-positive and 259 HIV-negative) demonstrated that exercising three to four times a week had a more protective effect than daily exercise.[52] Exercise in the HIV-positive group covered by this study showed an increase in CD4 count during a year by 7 percent. Some authors have reported that moderate training can be sustained without any substantial change in CD4 cell count.[53–55]

EXERCISE FOR THE MASSES

Aerobic exercise training is thus a promising nontoxic, nondrug adjunct therapy to improve physical fitness, increase quality of life, and potentially improve immune status (as indicated by reactivity to *Candida* skin test) of HIV-positive individuals. If it can be demonstrated that aerobic exercise increases anti-VIP/NTM antibodies in normal individuals (with the potential to decrease the risk of HIV transmission) and in HIV-positive individuals (with the potential to slow disease progression), it would strengthen the case that exercise can serve as a widely available and affordable intervention that is nontoxic and free of drug interactions. It would be applicable worldwide, in both developed and developing countries.

The Way Ahead

A SCIENTIFIC HYPOTHESIS RIDDLED WITH HOLES IS BEING
KEPT ALIVE BY VESTED INTERESTS REAPING HUGE PROFITS FROM
DRUGS AND VACCINES THAT ARE WORSE THAN USELESS,
WHILE SAFE AND EFFECTIVE APPROACHES BASED ON
NUTRITIONAL, HERBAL, AND OTHER LOW-COST, EASILY AVAILABLE
INTERVENTIONS ARE BEING SUPPRESSED AND IGNORED.

THERE IS AN URGENT NEED TO DEVELOP AND SUPPORT
EFFECTIVE, LOW-COST INTERVENTIONS TO COMBAT AIDS,
AND TO MAKE INFORMATION ON THE TOXICITY
OF ANTIRETROVIRAL DRUGS WIDELY AVAILABLE.

MEANWHILE, THERE SHOULD BE A GLOBAL MORATORIUM ON TRIALS
OF VACCINES ALREADY PROVEN INEFFECTIVE, AND A WIDE-RANGING,
OPEN DEBATE ON THE CAUSES AND CURES OF AIDS DISEASE.

GLOBAL INITIATIVE TO COMBAT AIDS BASED ON A DEEPLY FLAWED SCIENTIFIC HYPOTHESIS

Reports on the global "AIDS pandemic" were growing more alarming every day, as heroic multibillion-dollar global initiatives were being launched to combat it (see the first chapter).

We began our investigation with an open mind and a very modest goal: to review what is known about treating AIDS disease with traditional herbal medicines. Traditional herbal medicines are still the backbone of healthcare and are readily available in poor countries that have neither the access to expensive antiretroviral drugs nor the modern medical practitioners to administer them.

179

But as we proceeded, our curiosity and passion were aroused at every turn. A huge debate was raging around us, raising questions over every aspect of the "AIDS pandemic." Apparent answers led only to further questions, until we felt the need to unravel the disease epidemic thoroughly, from the basic science of what causes the disease to the politics of cure and prevention, which form an interconnected, interdependent whole.

We are astonished and dismayed at what we have uncovered. At the core of the multibillion-dollar global AIDS enterprise to provide cure and prevention for the suffering masses of humanity is a deeply flawed, unsupported scientific hypothesis about the cause of AIDS that has been protected from falsification for decades by the vested interests of the pharmaceutical industry and establishment scientists who gain prestige and research grants from promoting the flawed hypothesis.

THERE IS NO SUCH THING AS AN
AIDS DISEASE CAUSED BY HIV

"HIV causes AIDS. Curbing the spread of this virus must remain the first step towards eliminating this devastating disease." So said the Durban Declaration, as thousands were about to gather for the Thirteenth International AIDS Conference in July 2000 (see "AIDS and HIV"). The declaration, published in *Nature*, was signed by more than 5,000 people, among them Nobel laureates and directors of leading research institutions, scientific academies, and medical societies, such as the U.S. National Academy of Sciences, the Max Planck Institutes, the Pasteur Institute in Paris, the Royal Society of London, the AIDS society of India, and the National Institute of Virology in South Africa.

Yet even staunch defender of the "HIV causes AIDS" hypothesis Dr. Helene Gayle—then director of the U.S. Centers for Disease Control's National Center of HIV, STD, and TB Prevention, and now director of Bill and Melinda Gates Foundation's HIV, TB, and Reproductive Health Program—admitted at the end of the debate organized by South Africa's Presidential AIDS Advisory Panel that there is a general lack of standardization of the definition of AIDS throughout the world.

After fifteen years of research, there was no "gold standard" against which to measure the accuracy and reliability of the data generated from the commonly used methods to diagnose HIV infection; and the major task ahead was to develop such a golden standard. But it is still lacking to this day.

There are surrogate markers for the disease: circulating antibodies to HIV, viral proteins detected by Western blot, fragments of the HIV genome measured by polymerase chain reaction, and CD4 cell count. These are not only unreliable but are also poorly correlated with one another and with disease states (see "What is AIDS Disease?"). David Rasnick, an AIDS dissident scientist, sums up the situation: "These surrogate markers are causing a great deal of harm by labeling people with myriad diseases and conditions—even healthy people who only have antibodies to HIV—as having incurable AIDS, which is said to be invariably fatal. The surrogate markers are also being used to obtain FDA approval of clinically ineffective AIDS chemotherapies that are highly toxic and even lethal if taken long enough."[1]

WHAT IS AIDS DISEASE?

Peter Duesberg, David Rasnick, and Claus Koehnlein have argued that AIDS is a collection of chemical epidemics caused by recreational drugs, anti-HIV drugs, and malnutrition (see the chapter "AIDS and HIV").

Our investigations have borne this out. Not only recreational drugs, but also a whole range of "genotoxic" environmental agents may lead to AIDS disease, or something remarkably close to it, whether or not people are HIV-positive (see "HIV and Latent Viruses").

Shortly after the AIDS epidemics began in the United States and Europe, researchers found that illicit psychoactive and aphrodisiac drugs consumed in massive doses were the common factors and probable causes of AIDS. Drugs such as cocaine, heroin, nitrite inhalants, amphetamines, steroids, and lysergic acid (LSD) became widely available in the "drug explosion" during and after the Vietnam war, which coincided with the era of "gay liberation." Indeed, many AIDS researchers favored the hypothesis that drug use or "lifestyle" was the cause of AIDS well into the 1990s. But the mechanism whereby drug use leads to AIDS disease remains obscure to this day, mostly through lack of dedicated research.

There is also evidence to support the claim that most if not all HIV-positive individuals with no sign of AIDS disease would remain healthy if they avoided anti-HIV drugs like AZT and the newer HAART cocktails (see below), which have many toxic side effects, including death.

EXTREME POVERTY CAUSES AIDS

The figures for the global AIDS pandemic in Africa and elsewhere in the third world have been greatly inflated by redefining traditional diseases of the poor due to malnutrition and lack of drinkable water as AIDS (see "The African AIDS Epidemic" and "The Ugandan Success Story"). Nevertheless, there is a wasting disease characterized by AIDS, or acquired immune deficiency syndrome, with many causes, one of which, almost certainly, is extreme poverty.

South African President Thabo Mbeki came under fierce and sustained attack from the scientific establishment when he insisted that AIDS was linked to poverty and malnutrition and the collapse of the immune system. "The world's biggest killer and the greatest cause of ill health and suffering across the globe, including South Africa, is extreme poverty," he said in his speech to the Thirteenth International AIDS Conference in Durban, correctly diagnosing the 'poverty virus' they call HIV.[2]

There is now overwhelming scientific evidence that malnutrition and undernutrition associated with poverty compromise the immune system, leaving populations especially vulnerable to infection and disease (see "Eating Well for Health"). Protein–energy malnutrition (due to insufficient food) and a deficiency of a wide range of vitamins, co-factors, and minerals (due to intensive, industrial monoculture food-farming) all result in immune dysfunction. There is also growing evidence linking nutritional deficiencies with susceptibility to infection with HIV (or something like it) and progression to AIDS disease.

Results of the first clinical trials show that nutritional supplements can delay AIDS disease progression and death.

A trial of multivitamin supplement given to HIV-positive women in Tanzania, published in the *New England Journal of Medicine* in July 2004, gave the clearest indication that improving the nutritional status of HIV-positive women can delay disease progression and death (see "Eating Well Against HIV/AIDS").

A somewhat skeptical editorial in the journal written by two scientists involved in an antiretroviral treatment program in the third world called for a confirmation of the new findings and an evaluation of the effects of multivitamins in larger populations, while admitting, "As donor-funded initiatives expand in Africa, it has become clear that nutrition will have to be addressed in the treatment of HIV disease and AIDS."[3]

The editorial writers confessed that, in the focus-group discussions conducted before starting an antiretroviral treatment program in a large Nairobi slum, every group interviewed said the lack of food was the most likely cause of nonadherence to antiretroviral (ARV) drug therapy.

One focus group participant put it baldly, "If you give us ARVs, please give us food, just food."

The report of this trial raises a host of questions. Would the results of the trial have been even better if the women were given food in addition to multivitamin supplements? Could the women be suffering from protein–energy malnutrition and other micronutrient deficits? Why has it taken so long for vitamin supplements to be given? And why is food supplementation *still* not given to the women in this study, or indeed routinely given with ARVs?

SCANDAL OF THE GLOBAL INITIATIVES TO COMBAT AIDS

The answer is that the multibillion-dollar global initiatives to fight the AIDS pandemic are focusing on providing "cure" in the form of antiretroviral drugs, especially expensive brand-name drugs produced by big pharmaceutical companies in the United States (see "AIDS Aid: Big Profit for Pharma Giants"), and "prevention" in the form of candidate vaccines, massive trials of which are being carried out on populations in the third world (see "The Dangers of AIDS Vaccine Trials," "AIDS Vaccines, or Slow Bioweapons?" and "Controversy Breaks over AIDS Vaccine Trials").

The big scandal is that both the cure and the prevention are worse than useless. Hungry, vulnerable populations in the third world are thus being used as drug fodder for the pharmaceutical industry, and as guinea pigs to contribute knowledge to vaccine development, irrespective of efficacy and safety.

NO EVIDENCE THAT THE ANTI-HIV DRUGS WERE EFFECTIVE

There has never been evidence that the anti-HIV drugs are effective in treating AIDS. The licensing of the viral reverse transcriptase inhibitor

AZT, the first drug to be used in treating AIDS, was based on a study in 1987 showing that after four months of treatment, only one of 145 AIDS patients on AZT died, whereas 19 of 139 died in a control placebo group.

Among the survivors in the group of patients on AZT, however, thirty could be kept alive only with multiple blood transfusions. Also, many AZT recipients had developed life-threatening bone-marrow suppression and other symptoms that augured poorly for their future survival.

The newer drug cocktail, HAART, was no better. A front-page article in *The New York Times* in 1997 quoted Dr. Anthony Fauci, director of National Institutes of Allergy and Infectious Diseases as saying, "There is an increasing percentage of people in whom, after a period of time, the virus breaks through. People do quite well for six months, eight months or a year, and after a while, in a significant proportion, the virus starts to come back."[4]

The U.S. government finally set up an expert panel to review anti-HIV therapy in 2001, which led to recommendations to restrict the prescription of anti-HIV drugs and to delay treatment for the AIDS virus for as long as possible for people without symptoms, on account of the serious side effects. It is now routine for patients to take "holidays" from the toxic drug treatments when their markers of AIDS disease warrant it, and very few doctors would recommend long-term, uninterrupted anti-HIV drug treatment as a viable option.

As reviewed in detail in the chapter "Anti-HIV Drugs Do More Harm Than Good," although AZT given to HIV-positive pregnant women reduced the percentage of HIV-positive infants born, those children were 1.8 times more likely to develop severe disease, 2.4 times more likely to have severe immune suppression, and 3.2 times more likely to die than those born to HIV-positive mothers not taking AZT during pregnancy.

LONG-TERM HIV-POSITIVE SURVIVAL ASSOCIATED WITH NONUSE OF ANTIRETROVIRAL DRUGS

The AIDS research establishment has acknowledged the existence of long-term survivors of HIV infection as a "small minority" who show either no progression or slow progression to AIDS disease.

Many anecdotal reports and numerous scientific studies suggest that most long-term survivors have shunned antiviral drugs, and that use of antiretroviral drugs has led to quicker progression to AIDS. But these points are often understated in orthodox studies (see "Surviving and Thriving with HIV").

Claus Koehnlein in Kiel, Germany, initiated a study in 1985 of AIDS patients who had volunteered to abstain from anti-HIV treatments. Only three of thirty-six patients have died since their HIV antibodies were first detected, two of them sixteen years and one ten years after their first diagnosis of anti-HIV antibodies. *Most have recovered from their initial AIDS-indicator symptoms.*

By contrast, 63 percent of all German AIDS patients (11,700 out of 18,700), of which most were treated since 1987 with anti-HIV drugs, died during the same period.

There are contributing factors to long-term survival of HIV/AIDS other than shunning AZT/HAART, among them a strong natural immunity to HIV, avoidance of other high-risk activities such as drug-taking and unprotected sex, and taking control of one's life with optimism.

If all the evidence presented in this book is taken seriously, good nutrition, immunity-strengthening herbal medicines and supplements, probiotics, and exercise can all help delay disease progression (see below).

NO EFFECTIVE VACCINE BASED ON HIV/AIDS HYPOTHESIS

An effective vaccine against HIV has been the holy grail of the AIDS research establishment right from the moment HIV was identified as the "cause" of AIDS. That is just as misguided as the "cure."

Current vaccines are predominantly based on the HIV-1 envelope protein gp120, which, as a number of AIDS researchers have been warning for years, can harm the immune system of individuals in a number of ways, including overstimulating it, leaving it more vulnerable to subsequent infection and AIDS disease (see "The Dangers of AIDS Vaccine Trials" and "AIDS Vaccines, or Slow Bioweapons?"). There is emerging evidence that AIDS disease is characterized by an overstimulated, exhausted immune system, similar to that seen in aging (see "HIV and Latent Viruses" and "Eating Well for Health").

Also, the HIV gp120 gene has recombination hotspots similar to those in many viruses and bacteria and therefore has the potential to recombine with them to generate new deadly viruses and bacteria that can spread through the vaccinated populations and to wildlife (see "The Dangers of AIDS Vaccine Trials" and "AIDS Vaccines, or Slow Bioweapons?").

Despite that, companies and U.N. agencies have promoted these vaccines around the world in phase I and II and especially in large-scale phase III trials. The vaccines are now being tested in developing countries such as Thailand, South Africa, Uganda, and India, which have immunologically very vulnerable populations.

TRIALS OF INEFFECTIVE VACCINES ARE TO CONTRIBUTE TO VACCINE DEVELOPMENT

After a string of high-profile vaccine trial failures in which the candidate vaccines proved to be ineffective at best, and at worst unsafe, a fierce row has finally erupted in the pages of the journal *Science*, questioning the wisdom and ethics of continuing mass phase III trials in third world countries (see "Controversy Breaks over AIDS Vaccine Trials").

Dr. Dennis R. Burton of the Scripps Research Institute, La Jolla, California, and seventeen other signatories wrote, "We have concern about the wisdom of the U.S. government's sponsoring a recently initiated Phase III trial in Thailand. . . . Our opinion is that the overall approval process lacked input from independent immunologists and virologists, who could have judged whether the trial was scientifically meritorious. . . . As a whole, the scientific community must do a better job of bringing truly promising vaccine candidates to this stage of development and beyond."[5]

In reply, Dr. Robert Belshe of St. Louis University School of Medicine and twelve others stated, "Regardless of the specific vaccine efficacy, the trial still will make a substantial contribution to HIV vaccine research because we can apply what we learn to future vaccine candidates."[6]

In other words, the volunteers are being used as guinea pigs to contribute to HIV vaccine development, and neither the efficacy nor the safety is considered an issue.

VESTED INTERESTS DEPEND ON HIV BEING ACCEPTED AS THE SOLE CAUSE OF AIDS

Dr. Howard Urnovitz, another prominent AIDS dissident, has accused the signatories supporting the phase III trial of having vested interests that depend on the continued funding of HIV research and on HIV being accepted as the sole cause of AIDS. "Calling for the creation of a global AIDS vaccine enterprise in the midst of ongoing and widespread failure," he said, "rather than focusing on a cure for AIDS, seems a move to further enshrine the HIV concept, and those vested interests."[7]

Urnovitz also points out that Richard D. Klausner, former director of the National Cancer Institute (NCI)—from which the letter in support of the phase III trial was sent—is being investigated for receipt of personal payments from universities and research institutes to which the NCI awarded multimillion-dollar research grants during his tenure as director. Urnovitz calls upon the U.S. Congress to "open its eyes and investigate where AIDS money is going."

In September 2004, bad news came from another vaccine trial taking place in five countries and funded by the International AIDS Vaccine Initiative. Preliminary results from three countries—the United Kingdom, Kenya, and Uganda—showed that the vaccine had failed to elicit the critical immune response.[8] The editor of the *Lancet* pointed out that since 1987, there have been more than eighty trials of thirty different candidate AIDS vaccines, with no success in sight. He commented, "Contrary to the predictions and promises of most AIDS experts, the signs are that a vaccine to prevent HIV infection will not be found for, at the very least, several decades to come—if at all."[9]

It is clear that large vaccine companies are setting the agenda for trials. They construct their own scientific rationale for their studies. They also control the data generated, so that uncomfortable findings will not be subject to public scrutiny.

AIDS AND THE COMPLEXITY OF IMMUNITY

Evidence has emerged that AIDS is a disease of an overstimulated, exhausted immune system, rather like the "immunosenescence" found in the elderly, particularly those with poor nutritional status. Thus, immuno-stimulation through vaccination to prevent the disease is inappropriate and could make things worse.

Furthermore, genetic diversity and tissue compartmentalization are hallmarks of HIV-1 infection. A vaccine based on a single subtype is most likely to be ineffective; it could well be misdirected to the wrong tissue compartment and could make things worse through overstim-ulation of the immune system. The phenomenon of superinfection is pointing in that direction (see "Vaccinating People Against Their Own Genes").

It appears that some HIV-positive individuals who have success-fully suppressed the first strain of virus have no protection against a second (super-) infecting viral strain, even though a successful im-mune response to the original HIV strain is equivalent to a vacci-nation and should have protected them against the second infecting strain. Instead, if anything, these superinfected individuals dete-riorate much faster. This phenomenon is reminiscent of the "decep-tive imprinting" of the immune system in people given the gp120 vaccine, which rendered them vulnerable to subsequent infection by HIV.

More and more, it has become evident that a balanced type 1 and type 2 (cell-mediated and humoral) immune profile underlies success-ful long-term suppression of AIDS disease. The immune system works in close communication with other tissues and ultimately with all the organ systems. Especially well documented are the interaction of immune cells with the neurological and endocrine systems.

Psychoimmunology, the study of the physical influence of mind/emotion on the immune system, is now an established discipline that compels even the most reductionist scientists to adopt a more holistic perspective on health. It is not surprising, therefore, that long-term HIV survival is associated with the ability of individuals to take control of their own lives with optimism (see "Surviving and Thriving with HIV"), an association that needs to be much more thoroughly researched than it is.

The findings also suggest that a therapeutic approach to rebalancing the immune system is preferable to the use of toxic antiviral drugs.

AIDS AND THE FLUID GENOME

A mechanism whereby toxic drugs and environmental agents could cause AIDS has been pointed out by several AIDS researchers but has been completely ignored by the AIDS establishment (see "HIV and Latent Viruses").

Dr. Howard Urnovitz believes that HIV does not cause AIDS but is merely a marker for AIDS disease. He has proposed that AIDS is a "genomics disease." More specifically, HIV infection may wake up sleeping viruses hiding in the human genome, of which there are a great many, or it could recombine with the endogenous viruses to generate the killer viruses.

In fact, HIV may not be a virus at all but rather one among many circulating species of RNAs in disease states, which consist of bits of human genome sequences scrambled and spliced together, probably through the action of mobile genetic elements. These mobile genetic elements become activated through inflammatory responses induced by tissue injury, toxic chemical agents, radiation, or infectious agents. This could account for many other chronic diseases, such as Gulf War Syndrome and mad cow disease, according to Urnovitz.[10]

Yet another connection to a latent virus lurking in the human genome was made in the 1990s. Dr. Konnie Knox and Dr. Donald Carrigan in the Medical College of Wisconsin, Milwaukee, found evidence of human herpes virus (HHV-6) infection in 100 percent of HIV-positive patients, even before the onset of AIDS disease. Knox and Carrigan also found HHV-6 infections in people who had died of AIDS-like symptoms and who were HIV-negative.[11]

HHV-6 is present in some 90 percent of the general population, and there is already a wide spectrum of ailments attributed to it. In immune-suppressed patients, this includes fever, hepatitis, failure of bone marrow engraftment, encephalitis, and interstitial pneumonitis. In immuno-competent adults, HHV-6 has been linked to infectious mononucleosis, autoimmune disorders, chronic fatigue syndrome, fulminant hepatitis, non-Hodgkin's lymphomas, and Hodgkin's disease.

HHV-6 is a member of the herpes virus family and is closely related to human cytomegalovirus. Like other members of this family, it causes a primary infection and then can establish latent infection for the lifetime of the infected host, often by integrating into the genome of the host cells. They become activated in immune suppression or, very possibly, by toxic chemicals and other environmental insults.

If any or all of these theories are correct, vaccinating against HIV may indeed be vaccinating people against their own genes, risking autoimmune disease; or worse, it could scramble gene sequences through the inflammatory immune response and wake up killer viruses lurking in the genome.

ALTERNATIVE APPROACHES TO PREVENTION

Our investigations also uncovered a plethora of alternative approaches to prevention and therapy that are being suppressed or not followed up by dedicated research.

Away from the glare of acrimonious debate, independent as well as independent-minded scientists have quietly adopted a different approach to vaccine development (see "The 'Pink Panacea': An AIDS Vaccine?"). A company based in Thailand has developed an oral vaccine against HIV/AIDS. The makers of a pink pill called V1 claim striking success in the treatment of HIV/AIDS symptoms. V1 is said to be a therapeutic vaccine comprising "HIV antigens from pooled clinical isolates from HIV infected donors." V1 works on the premise that HIV/AIDS is a disease of mucosal immunity, so targeting antigens at mucosal surfaces is a valid clinical approach. It has broad-spectrum activity against many HIV subtypes and is stable in ambient tropical temperatures for three years, making refrigeration unnecessary. And no special skills or syringes are needed to administer the pill.

NUTRITIONAL THERAPY

The first successful trial of multivitamin supplementation in delaying AIDS progression and death in HIV-positive subjects (see "Eating Well Against HIV/AIDS") has come in the wake of a wealth of evidence linking malnutrition and undernutrition with a range of immune deficiencies that leave populations vulnerable to infection and disease, including AIDS (see "Eating Well for Health").

Support for nutritional cause of disease and health is found in the impressive correlation between the prevalence of HIV/AIDS, other viral infections, and cancer with selenium-poor soil, in Africa and in China; and the claimed successes of selenium and antioxidant supplement in the treatment of AIDS (see "Selenium Conquers AIDS").

No discussion on nutrition today is complete without mentioning probiotics, beneficial bacteria that inhabit the gut mucosa and provide numerous essential metabolic, detoxifying, and immune services to keep the host well nourished and free from infection (see the chapters "Eating Well for Health" and "Probiotics for Life After HIV/AIDS").

TRADITIONAL HERBAL THERAPIES

A cornucopia of immune-boosting and healing biochemicals are found in traditional medicinal plants that have been used by people in all cultures for millennia.

Traditional medicinal plants and their complex carbohydrates are increasingly found to be effective immune boosters (see "Herbs for Immunity"). Since 40 percent of the global total of HIV/AIDS cases live in Asian countries with a rich tradition of herbal medicines, it is essential that these people be provided with accessible conventional therapies as well as herbal alternatives that are indigenous to their healing traditions.

In Africa, traditional medicine (TM) is used by up to 80 percent of the population to meet primary healthcare needs and is crucial in the fight against infectious diseases. The ratio of conventional, or Western-trained, general practitioners to patients is 1:20,000, whereas the availability of TM practitioners is 1:200 to 1:400. This highlights the need for reliable and affordable herbal medicines that are locally available. Among the many medicinal herbs used in treating different symptoms attributed to AIDS disease, *Sutherlandia* has emerged as being especially successful. It has been approved by the Indigenous Knowledge Systems Division of the Medical Research Council in South Africa.

An ancient common weed, St. John's wort (*Hypericum*), widely used for treating depression, has caught the attention of the AIDS community (see "*Hypericum* Versus HIV/AIDS"). *In vitro* studies of plant extracts and limited clinical trials have been conducted after encouraging anecdotal reports from doctors.

Powerful extracts from fungi are bridging the gap between traditional and conventional treatments of cancer and HIV/AIDS (see "Therapeutic Mushrooms") in the form of "host defense potentiators," long-chain sugar polymers that somehow prime the immune system. These are beneficial adjuncts for people undergoing chemotherapy for cancer or acupuncture and traditional Chinese medicine for HIV/AIDS.

Older approved drugs—such as warfarin, cimetidine, levamisole, acetaminophen, and gramicidin—could also make a cheap and safe alternative to current anti-HIV drug cocktails (see "AIDS Therapy from Cheap Generics").

EXERCISE AGAINST HIV/AIDS

Evidence is emerging on how exercise may help treat and prevent AIDS. If so, the simplest, most widely available and affordable natural "vaccine" is being ignored (see "Exercise Versus AIDS"). If an Achilles' heel exists in HIV, it might be in the central portion of gp120 (residues 280–302, designated as peptide NTM). This portion of the molecule is highly conserved in all known HIV variants and appears to be crucial for viral infectivity. Unfortunately, this part of gp120 is not immunogenic in humans because the immune system treats it as "self," possibly due to peptide NTM's similarity to several human proteins. An antibody to vasoactive intestinal peptide (VIP), however, which is found in both HIV-positive and HIV-negative individuals, seems to have reactivity to this region of the gp120 molecule.

Thus increase in circulating VIP can counteract the effects of the HIV gp120 by overcoming the latter's inhibition of NK cells, and by stimulating the production of VIP autoantibodies, which can also bind gp120 and prevent it from binding to NK cells. It appears that exercise increases VIP and antibodies to VIP. Also, VIP and the peptide NTM may be responsible for the interaction between HIV and the CD4 receptor, which represents the first step in the process of infection. So an increase in VIP could also block HIV infection directly.

RECOMMENDATIONS

Based on the evidence presented in this book, we recommend that the following actions be taken as a matter of urgency.

➥ Effective, low-cost interventions to combat AIDS should be made widely available to all. In particular, measures should be taken to provide adequate nutrition and to overcome lack of food and other nutritional deficiencies in AIDS patients. Traditional medicinal interventions should be made accessible to treat specific AIDS-defining symptoms.

➥ Treatment with toxic antiretroviral drugs should be delayed for as long as possible, in line with guidelines already in place in the United States, and information on the toxicity of antiretroviral drugs should be made widely available and accessible.

➥ There should be a global moratorium on trials of vaccines already proven ineffective.

➥ Support for research and development of many low-cost, safe, and effective interventions to combat AIDS should be greatly increased at the expense of antiretroviral drugs and vaccines in the current global initiatives to combat AIDS.

➥ There should be an open, wide-ranging debate on the causes of and cures for AIDS disease.

References

AIDS: A GLOBAL PANDEMIC

1. UNAIDS. AIDS Epidemic Update, December 0003.
2. JP Gutierrez, B Johns, T Adam, et al. "Achieving the WHO/UNAIDS antiviral treatment 3 by 5 goal: What will it cost?" *Lancet* 364 (2004): 63–4.
3. S Boseley. "AIDS defeating world's best efforts as record numbers are infected." *The Guardian*, 7 July 2004.
4. W Brummer. "SA's AIDS figures '33% lower.'" News 24, 6 July 2004. www.news24.com/News24/South_Africa/AIDS_Focus/0,,2-7-659_1553748,00.html
5. S Shacinda. "U.S. needs good plan to give AIDS funds—health chief." 1 December 2003. www.alertnet.org/thenews/newsdesk/5596293.htm
6. "New drug plan marks World AIDS Day." *Taipei Times*, 2 December 2003.
7. "Bush's budget undermines AIDS Fight—Africa action." *Accra Mail*, 9 February 2004. www.allAfrica.com (subscription required).

WHAT IS AIDS DISEASE?

1. Centers for Disease Control and Prevention. "1993 Revised Classification System for HIV Infection and Expanded Surveillance Case Definition for AIDS Among Adolescents and Adults." *Morbidity and Mortality Weekly Report* 41 (1992): 1–19.
2. D Rasnick. "HIV antibody test is the Achilles heel of AIDS Inc." Rapid Responses to News Extra: D Spurgeon, "Canadian aboriginals in Vancouver face AIDS epidemic." *British Medical Journal* 326 (2003): 126e.
3. Ibid.
4. C Johnson. "Whose antibodies are they anyway? Factors known to cause false positive HIV antibody test results." *Continuum* (London) 4 (no. 3, September/October 1996): 4–5.
5. Presidential AIDS Advisory Panel Report, a synthesis report of the deliberations by the panel of experts invited by the President of the Republic of South Africa, the Honourable Mr. Thabo Mbeki, March 2001.
6. D Rasnick. "An abuse of surrogate markers for AIDS." Rapid Responses to News Extra: D Spurgeon, "Canadian aboriginals in Vancouver face AIDS epidemic." *British Medical Journal* 326 (2003), 126e.
7. M Seligman, DA Warrell, J-P Aboulker, et al. "Concorde: MRC/ANRS randomised double-blind controlled trial of immediate and deferred zidovudine in symptom-free HIV infection." *Lancet* 343 (1994): 871–81.
8. TR Fleming, DL DeMets. "Surrogate end points in clinical trials: Are we being misled?" *Annals of Internal Medicine* 125 (1996): 605–13.
9. MA Sande, CC Carpenter, CG Cobbs, et al. "Antiretroviral therapy for adult HIV-infected patients: Recommendations from a state-of-the-art conference."

National Institute of Allergy and Infectious Diseases state-of-the-art panel on anti-retroviral therapy for adult HIV-infected patients. *Journal of the American Medical Association* 270 (1993): 2583–9.

10. TR Fleming. "Surrogate markers in AIDS and cancer trials." *Statistics in Medicine* 13 (1994): 1423–35.

11. DH Schwartz, OB Laeyendecker, S Arango-Jaramillo, et al. "Extensive evaluation of a seronegative participant in an HIV-1 vaccine trial as a result of false-positive PCR." *Lancet* 350 (1997): 256–9.

12. C Defer, H Agut, A Garbarg-Chenon, et al. "Multicentre quality control of polymerase chain reaction [viral load] for detection of HIV DNA." *AIDS* 6 (1992): 659–63.

13. MP Busch, DR Henrard, IK Hewlett, et al. "Poor sensitivity, specificity, and reproducibility of detection of HIV-1 DNA in serum by polymerase chain reaction." *Journal of Acquired Immune Deficiency* 5 (1992): 872–7.

14. Rasnick, "HIV antibody test."

AIDS AND HIV

1. Medical Encyclopedia, MedlinePlus, updated 12 June 2002.

2. PH Duesberg. "Retroviruses as carcinogens and pathogens: Expectations and reality." *Cancer Research* 47 (1987): 1199–1220.

3. P Duesberg, C Koehnlein, D Rasnick. "The chemical bases of the various AIDS epidemics: Recreational drugs, anti-viral therapy and malnutrition." *Journal of Biosciences* 28 (2003): 383–412.

4. Durban Declaration. *Nature* 406 (2000): 15–16.

5. GT Stewart, S Mhlongo, E de Harven, et al. "The Durban Declaration is not accepted by all." *Nature* 407 (2000): 286.

6. Presidential AIDS Advisory Panel Report, a synthesis report of the deliberations by the panel of experts invited by the President of the Republic of South Africa, the Honourable Mr. Thabo Mbeki, March 2001.

7. GM Oppenheimer. "Causes, cases and cohorts: The role of epidemiology in the historical construction of AIDS," in E Fee and DM Fox, editors, *AIDS: The Making of a Chronic Disease*. Berkeley, CA: University of California Press, 1992, 49–83.

8. C Mims, DO White. *Viral Pathogenesis and Immunology*. Oxford: Blackwell, 1984.

9. M Seligmann, L Chess, JL Fahey, et al. "AIDS: An immunologic reevaluation." *New England Journal of Medicine* 311 (1984): 1286–92.

10. Duesberg et al., op. cit.

11. DD Ho. "Time to hit HIV, early and hard." *New England Journal of Medicine* 333 (1995): 450–1.

12. Italian Register for HIV Infection in Children. "Rapid disease progression in HIV-1 perinatally infected children born to mothers receiving zidovudine monotherapy during pregnancy." *AIDS* 13 (1999): 927–33.

13. "U.S. panel seeks changes in treatment of AIDS virus." L Altman, *New York Times*, 4 February 2001.

14. Duesberg et al., op. cit.

THE AFRICAN AIDS EPIDEMIC

1. *World Health Organisation Weekly Epidemiological Record* no. 10, 7 March 1986, p. 71.
2. CF Gilks. "What use is a clinical case definition for AIDS in Africa?" *British Medical Journal* 303 (9 November 1991): 1189–90.
3. T Bethell. "Inventing an epidemic: The traditional diseases of Africa are called AIDS." *American Spectator*, April 2000.
4. J Jerndal. "Smoke and mirrors: The great illusionist number called AIDS statistics." *Health Counter News*, Easter 2002.
5. Peter H Duesberg. *Infectious AIDS: Have We Been Misled?* Berkeley, CA: North Atlantic Books, 1995.
6. E Papadopulos-Eleopulos, VF Turner, JM Papadimitrious, et al. "AIDS in Africa: Distinguishing fact and fiction." *World Journal of Microbiology and Biotechnology* 11 (1995): 135–43.
7. Bethell, op. cit.
8. C Geshetker. "A critical reappraisal of African AIDS research and Western sexual stereotypes." Prepared for Presentation to General Assembly Meeting, Council for the Development of Social Science Research in Africa (CODESRIA), Dakar, Senegal, 14–18 December 1998, revised 5 May 1999.
9. www.worldbank.org/afr/aids/overview.htm
10. C Denny. "Brown and Bono appeal for doubling of aid cash." *The Guardian*, 17 February 2004.
11. *Corporate Watch* newsletter, no. 6, April–May 2002.
12. MW Ho. "Ethiopia to feed herself." *Science in Society* 16 (Autumn 2002).
13. J Wise, K Mistry, S Reid. "Neuropsychiatric complications of nevirapine treatment." *British Medical Journal* 324 (13 April 2002): 879.
14. G Mahoney. "Interview: David Rasnick, Out of Africa." *San Francisco Herald*, October 2000. www.virusmyth.net/aids/data/gminterviewdr.htm
15. Quoted in N Hodgkinson, "Cry, beloved country: How Africa became the victim of a non-existent epidemic of HIV/AIDS." www.virusmyth.net/aids/data/nhcry.htm

THE UGANDAN SUCCESS STORY

1. D Rasnick. "HIV/AIDS is indeed a colossal catastrophe." *British Medical Journal* rapid response to L Stabinski, K Pelley, S T Jacob, et al., "Reframing HIV and AIDS," *British Medical Journal* 327 (2003): 1101–3.
2. World Health Organization. "Global situation of the HIV/AIDS pandemic, end 2001. Part 1." *Weekly Epidemiological Record* 76 (2001): 381–4.
3. Rasnick, op. cit.
4. J Parkhurst. "The crisis of AIDS and the politics of response: The case of Uganda." *International Relations of the Asia-Pacific* 15 (2001): 69–87.
5. Government of Uganda, Uganda AIDS Commission, UNAIDS. "The national strategic framework for HIV/AIDS activities in Uganda: 2000/1–2005/6."
6. Parkhurst, "Crisis of AIDS."
7. Rasnick, op. cit.

8. JO Parkhurst. "The Ugandan success story? Evidence and claims of HIV-1 prevention." *Lancet* 360 (2002): 78–80.
9. Parkhurst, "Ugandan Success Story."
10. C Wendo. "AIDS figures slashed." *New Vision* (Kampala), 22 July 2004. www.allafrica.com/stories/200407220096.html (subscription required).

AIDS AID: BIG PROFIT FOR PHARMA GIANTS

1. S. Boseley. "AIDS defeating world's best efforts as record numbers are infected." *The Guardian*, 7 July 2004.
2. S. Boseley. "US firms try to block cheap AIDS drugs." *The Guardian*, 20 March 2004.
3. "Study says generic anti-HIV drugs meet U.S. standards." *Advocate*, 22 April 2004. www.advocate.com/new_news.asp?id=12151&sd=04/22/04
4. "Third World pharma companies unapologetic about cloning anti-HIV drugs." *Lifestyle News*, 2 July 2004. news.lifestyle.co.uk/health/15767-health.htm
5. Boseley, "AIDS defeating world's best efforts."
6. Boseley, "US firms try to block cheap AIDS drugs."
7. "World Trade Organisation generic drug deal not being implemented, leaving developing countries without antivirals, UNAIDS says." Henry J. Kaiser Family Foundation, 4 July 2004. www.kaisernetwork.org/daily_reports/rep_hiv.cfm
8. AM Bwomezi. "How US is turning AIDS into big business." *The Monitor* (Kampala), 20 July 2004. allafrica.com/stories/200407200500.html (subscription required).
9. Ibid.
10. Ibid.
11. Ibid.
12. K Kumara. "India adopts WTO patent law with Left Front support." World Socialist Web Site, 16 April 2005. www.wsws.org/articles/2005/apr2005/indi-a16.shtml

ANTI-HIV DRUGS DO MORE HARM THAN GOOD

1. P Duesberg, C Koehnlein, D Rasnick. "The chemical bases of the various AIDS epidemics: Recreational drugs, anti-viral therapy and malnutrition." *Journal of Biosciences* 28 (2003): 383–412.
2. D Rasnick. "Do AIDS drugs deserve credit for extending life?" Responses to News Extra: David Spurgeon, "Canadian aboriginals in Vancouver face AIDS epidemic." *British Medical Journal* 326 (2003): 126e.
3. Centers for Disease Control and Prevention. "U.S. HIV and AIDS cases reported through December 1997," year-end edition. *HIV AIDS Surveillance Report* 9 (no. 2, 1997): 1–43.
4. Centers for Disease Control and Prevention. "1993 revised classification system for HIV infection and expanded surveillance case definition for AIDS among adolescents and adults." *Morbidity and Mortality Weekly Report* 41 (1992): 1–19.
5. JA Levy. "Caution: Should we be treating HIV infection early?" *Lancet* 352 (1998): 982–3.

6. J-P Viard, M Burgard, J-B Hubert, et al. "Impact of 5 years of maximally successful highly active antiviral therapy on CD4 cell count and HIV-1 DNA level." *AIDS* 18 (2004): 45–9.

7. C Chesson. "NIH smart drugs study (6000 patients) on the efficacy of structured treatment interruptions for HIV" (part 11 of 15). *Journal of Immunity* 2 (2004): 2. www.keephope.net/j2004v2n2.html

8. Ibid.

9. Ibid.

10. AIDS Community Research Initiative of America. "Viread." *ACRIA Update* 12 (no. 4, Fall 2003); 13 (no. 1, Winter 2004). www.acria.org/treatment/treatment_edu_fall03-win04update_tdf.html

11. DD Richman, SC Morton, T Wrin, et al. "The prevalence of antiretroviral drug resistance in the United States." *AIDS* 18 (no. 10, 2004): 393–401.

12. "Ten per cent of AIDS patients resistant to drugs." *International Herald Tribune*, 17 July 2003.

13. Durban Declaration. *Nature* 406 (2000): 15–16.

14. DD Richman, MA Fischl, MH Crieco, et al. "The toxicity of azidothymidine (AZT) in the treatment of patients with AIDS and AIDS-related complex." *New England Journal of Medicine* 317 (1987): 192–7.

15. MA Fischl, DD Richman, MH Grieco, et al. "The efficicacy of azidothymidine (AZT) in the treatment of patients with AIDS and AIDS-related complex." *New England Journal of Medicine* 317 (1987): 185–91.

16. MH Walker. *Dirty Medicine: Science, Big Business and the Assault on Natural Health Care*. London: Slingshot Publications, 1994. E-book available at www.truthcampaign.ukf.net/mainpages/dirtymedicine.html

17. M Seligman, DA Warrell, J-P Aboulker, et al. "Concorde: MRC/ANRS randomised double-blind controlled trial of immediate and deferred zidovudine in symptom-free HIV infection." *Lancet* 343 (1994): 871–81.

18. SG Stolberg. "1997 Year of the crash: Despite new AIDS drugs, many still lose the battle." *New York Times*, 22 August 1997.

19. Rasnick, op. cit.

20. Centers for Disease Control and Prevention. "U.S. HIV and AIDS cases reported through December 1997," year-end edition. *HIV AIDS Surveillance Report* 9 (no. 2, 1997): 1–43.

21. RB Reisler, C Han, WJ Burman, et al. "Grade 4 events are as important as AIDS events in the era of HAART." *Journal of Acquired Immune Deficiency Syndromes* 34 (2003): 379–86.

22. EM Conner, RS Spreling, R Gelber, et al. "Reduction of maternal-infant transmission of human immunodeficiency virus type 1 with zidovudine treatment." *New England Journal of Medicine* 331 (1994): 1173–80.

23. Italian Register for HIV Infection in Children. "Rapid disease progression in HIV-1 perinatally infected children born to mothers receiving zidovudine monotherapy during pregnancy." *AIDS* 13 (1999): 927–33.

24. RS de Souza, O Gómez-Marin, GB Scott, et al. "Effect of prenatal zidovudine on disease progression in perinatally HIV-1–infected infants." *Journal of Acquired Immune Deficiency Syndromes* 24 (2000): 154–61.

25. S Blanche, M Tardieu, P Rustin, et al. "Persistent mitochondrial dysfunction and perinatal exposure to antiretroviral nucleoside analogues." *Lancet* 354 (1999): 1084–9.

26. M Culane, MG Fowler, SS Lee, et al. "Lack of long term effects of in utero exposure to zidovudine among uninfected children born to HIV-infected women." *Journal of the American Medical Association* 281 (1999): 151–7.

27. Duesberg et al., op. cit.

28. Ibid.

29. Ibid.

30. Ibid.

31. Robert Koch Institute. "2000 HIV/AIDS-Halbjahresbericht I/2000." *Epidemiology Bulletin* 15 (September 2000): 1–16.

SURVIVING AND THRIVING WITH HIV

1. L Altman. "Long-term survivors may hold key clues to puzzle of AIDS." *New York Times*, 24 January 1995. Cited in "Long-Time Survivors," compiled by Bill Wells. heal_portland.tripod.com/long.htm

2. J McMenamin, et al. "Clinical progression of HIV in the Glenochil prison cohort." *HIV in Clinical Practice*, abstract O18, Cambridge, 1995. Cited at www.aidsmap.com/en/docs/7B3DE4F7-E272-405D-A473-9F75E14CDF15.asp

3. J Guerin, et al. "Nonprogressors in the Australian long-term nonprogressor cohort: Proportions and predictors." Second International AIDS Society Conference on HIV Pathogenesis and Treatment, Paris, abstract 454, 2003. Cited at www.aidsmap.com/en/docs/81D8E0F6-BB5A-43E1-A0C8-5D40F71D6BAF.asp

4. T Harrer, E Harrer, SA Kalams, et al. "Strong cytotoxic T-cell and weak neutralizing antibody responses in a subset of persons with stable nonprogressing HIV type-1 infection." *AIDS Research and Human Retroviruses* 12 (1996): 585. Cited in "Long-Time Survivors," compiled by Bill Wells. heal_portland.tripod.com/long.htm

5. P Duesberg, D Rasnick. "The drugs-AIDS hypothesis." *Continuum*, February/March 1997. www.virusmyth.net/aids/data/pddrdrugaids.htm

6. Ibid.

7. T Hand. "Why antiviral drugs cannot resolve AIDS." *Reappraising AIDS* 4 (9 September 1996). Cited in Duesberg and Rasnick, op. cit.

8. A Munoz. "Disease progression: 15 percent of HIV-infected men will be long-term survivors." *AIDS Weekly*, 15 May 1995, 3–4; 29 May 1995, 5–6. Cited in Duesberg and Rasnick, op. cit.

9. G Pantaleo, F Menzo, M Vaccarezza, et al. "Studies in subjects with long-term nonprogressive human immunodeficiency infection." *New England Journal of Medicine* 332 (1995): 2091–6.

10. S Buchbinder, MH Katz, N Hessol, et al. "Long-term HIV-1 infection without immunologic progression." *AIDS* 8 (1994): 1123. Cited in Duesberg and Rasnick, op. cit.

11. M Tanaka. "Abrams cautious on use of new AIDS drugs." *Synapse: The University of California-San Francisco Student Newspaper* (10 October 1996). Cited in "Long-Time Survivors," compiled by Bill Wells. heal_portland.tripod.com/long.htm

12. Y Cao, L Quin, L Zhang, et al. "Virologic and immunologic characterization of long-term survivors of HIV- type 1 infection." *New England Journal of Medicine* 332 (26 January 1995): 201–8.

13. T Simmons. "Living on the edge." *The Advocate*, 5 December 1995. Cited in Duesberg and Rasnick, op. cit.

14. "Leoutsakas appointed to national CDC position." www.salisbury.edu/newsevents/pressrel/archives/2004/041904LA.asp

15. M. Callen. *Surviving AIDS*. New York: HarperCollins, 1990, 23. Cited in Duesberg and Rasnick, op. cit.

16. The Toronto Survey on Complementary Therapies. Palliser Health Authority, September 1996. Cited in J Castro, "Study of long term survivors proves to be useless." *Continuum* 4, no. 4, 1999. www.garynull.com/Documents/Continuum/StudyLongTermSurvivorsProvesToBeUseless.htm

THE DANGERS OF AIDS VACCINE TRIALS

1. "Global Investment and Expenditures on Preventive HIV Vaccines: Methods and Results for 2002." Working Draft 7 July 2004, International AIDS Vaccine Initiative. www.iavi.org/pdf/Global%20Investment%20Expenditure%20HIV%20Vaccines%202002.pdf

2. J Prljic, N Veljković, T Doliana, et al. "Identificaion of an active Chi recombinational hot spot within the HIV-1 envelope gene: Consequences for development of AIDS vaccine." *Vaccine* 17 (1999): 1462–7.

3. "Superviruses and superbugs from AIDS vaccines." *ISIS News* 9/10 (July 2001). www.i-sis.org.uk/isisnews/i-sisnews9-11.php

4. MW Ho. "How to keep in concert." Institute of Science and Society report, 9 September 2004. www.i-sis.org.uk/KeepingInConcert.php

5. J Prljic et al., op.cit.

6. F Simo, P Mauclere, P Roques, et al. "Identification of a new human immunodeficiency virus type I distinct from group M and group O." *Nature Medicine* 4 (1998): 1032–7.

7. V Veljković, et al. "Safety and Ethical Considerations of AIDS Vaccines," Chapter 7. (Courtesy of Dr. Veljković.)

8. "The HIV vaccine paradox." *Science* 15 (1994): 475.

9. CP Locher, RM Grant, T Wrin, et al. "Antibody and cellular immune responses in breakthrough infection subject after HIV type 1 glycoprotein 120 vaccination." *AIDS Research and Human Retoviruses* 71 (1999): 1685.

10. "Massive trial of AIDS vaccine to begin in Thailand." CNN Interactive, 10 February 1999. www.cnn.com/HEALTH/9902/10/aids.vaccine.trial

11. D Gold. "IAVI launches project to develop oral HIV vaccine." *IAVI Report*, April–June 2000.

12. IJ Caley, MR Betts, DM Irlbeck, et al. "Humoral, mucosal, and cellular immunity in response to a human immunodeficiency virus type 1 immunogen expressed by a Venezuelan equine encephalitis virus vaccine vector." *Journal of Virology* 71 (1997): 3031.

13. "SA to conduct AIDS vaccine trials." *About South Africa Health*, June 23, 2003.

14. Caley et al., op. cit.

15. CG Murphy, WT Lucas, RE Means, et al. "Vaccine protection against simian immunodeficiency virus by recombinant strains of herpes simplex virus." *Journal of Virology* 74 (2000): 7745.

16. "New Preventative Technology: Providing New Options to Stop the Spread of HIV/AIDS." AIDS Vaccines: An R&D Briefing. International AIDS Vaccines Initiative, Dublin, Ireland, 24 June 2004.

17. "Preventative AIDS vaccine candidates in human clinical trials." International AIDS Vaccine Initiative. www.iavi.org/viewfile.cfm?fid=377

18. O Picard, J Lebas, JC Imbert, et al. "Complications of intramuscular/subcutaneous immune therapy in severely immune-compromised individuals." *Journal of Acquired Immune Deficiency Syndromes* 4 (1991): 641.

19. V Yusibov, A Modelska, K Steplwski, et al. "Antigens produced in plants by infection with chimeric plant viruses immunize against rabies virus and HIV-1." *Proceedings of the National Academy of Sciences U.S.A.* 94 (1997): 5784.

20. R Gernandez-Larsson. "Eat your corn flakes—and get vaccinated?" *AIDScience* 2 (no. 7, April 2002). www.aidscience.com/Articles/aidscience019.asp

21. Reviewed in MW Ho, A Ryan, J Cummins. "Hazards of transgenic plants with the CaMV 35S promoter." *Microbial Ecology in Health and Disease* 12 (2000): 6–11.

22. MJ Gibbs, GF Weiller. "Evidence that a plant virus switched hosts to infect a vertebrate and then recombined with a vertebrate-infected virus." *Proceedings of the National Academy of Sciences U.S.A.* 96 (1999): 8022.

23. "New guidelines on ethics of HIV vaccine research issued." HealthL. Health Systems Trust 2000-03-16. www.hst.org.za/news/20000322

AIDS VACCINES, OR SLOW BIOWEAPONS?

1. P Cohen. "AIDS vaccine trial is abandoned by the US." *New Scientist*, 9 March 2002, 14. www.newscientist.com/article.ns?id=mg17323331.700 (subscription required)

2. SL Buge, H-L Ma, RR Amara, et al. "Gp120-alum boosting of a Gag-Pol-Env DNA/MVA AIDS vaccine: Higher pre challenge antibody but poorer control of a live viral challenge." *AIDS Research and Human Retroviruses* 19 (2003): 891–900.

3. H Köhler, S Müller, V Veljković. "No hope for an AIDS vaccine soon." *AIDScience* 2 (no. 5, March 2002). aidscience.org/Articles/aidscience018.asp

4. JW Shiver, T-M Fu, L Chen, et al. "Replication-incompetent adenoviral vaccine vector elicits effective anti-immunodeficiency-virus immunity." *Nature* 415 (2002): 331–4.

5. Ibid.

6. L Garrett. "Skeptical about AIDS vaccine: Testing method questioned." *Newsday* (New York), 6 September 2001.

7. DH Barouch, J Kunstman, MJ Kuroda, et al. "Eventual AIDS vaccine failure in a rhesus monkey by viral escape from cytotoxic T lymphocytes." *Nature* 415 (2002): 335–9.

8. S Gandon, MJ Mackinnon, S Nee, et al. "Imperfect vaccines and the evolution of pathogen virulence." *Nature* 414 (2001): 751–5.

9. R Gernandez-Larsson. "Eat your corn flakes—and get vaccinated?" *AIDScience* 2 (no. 7, April 2002). www.aidscience.com/Articles/aidscience019.asp

10. V Veljković, MW Ho. "Edible AIDS vaccine or dangerous biological agent?" *AIDScience* 2 (no. 7, April 2002). www.aidscience.com/Debates/aidscience019d.asp

11. SN Shchelkunov, RK Salyaev, NI Rekoslavskaya, et al. "The obtaining of transgenic tomato plant producing chimerical proteins TBI-HbsAg." *Doklady Biochemistry and Biophysics* 396 (2004): 139–42.

12. SN Shchelkunov, RK Salyaev, NI Rekoslavskaya, et al. "The obtaining of transgenic tomato plant producing chimerical proteins TBI-HbsAg" (Russian). *Doklady Biochemistry* 396 (May–June 2004): 139–42.

13. CA Rinzler. "The ultimate health food." *New York Daily News*, 7 July 2004. www.nydailynews.com/city_life/health/story/209617p-180648c.html

14. "VaxGen Announces Initial Results of its Phase III AIDS Vaccine Trial." VaxGen Press Release, 24 February 2003. www.vaxgen.com/pressroom/index.html

15. V Veljković, S Müller, H Köhler. "Does VaxGen hide the breakthrough infections?" *Lancet* 361 (2003): 1743.

16. MW Ho. "AIDS vaccine trials dangerous." *ISIS Report* (29 July 2001). www.i-sis.org.uk/AIDS_virus.php

17. PW Berman, AM Gray, T Wrin, et al. "Genetic and immunologic characterization of virus infecting MN-rgp120-vaccinated volunteers." *Journal of Infectious Disease* 176 (1997): 384–97.

18. RI Connor, BT Korber, BS Graham, et al. "Immunological and virological analysis of persons infected by human immunodeficiency virus type 1 while participating in trials of recombinant gp120 subunit vaccines." *Journal of Virology* 72 (1998): 1552–76.

19. CP Locher, RM Grant, EA Collisson, et al. "Antibody and cellular immune responses in breakthrough infection subjects after HIV type 1 glycoprotein 120 vaccination." *AIDS Research and Human Retroviruses* 71 (1999): 1685–759.

20. H Kohler, PL Nara, S Muller. "Deceptive imprinting in the immune response to HIV-1 infection." *Immunology Today* 15 (1994): 475–8.

21. V Veljković, R Metlaš, H Köhler, et al. "AIDS epidemic at the beginning of the third millennium: Time for a new AIDS vaccine strategy." *Vaccine* 19 (2001): 1855–62.

22. R Metlaš, V Veljković. "Does HIV-1 gp120 manipulate human immune network?" *Vaccine* 13 (1995): 355–9.

23. R Metlaš, D Trajkovic, T Srdic, et al. "Anti-V3 and anti-IgG antibodies of healthy individuals share complementarity structures." *Journal of AIDS* 21 (1999): 266–70.

24. R Metlaš, D Trajkovic, T Srdic, et al. "Human immunodeficiency virus V3 peptide-reactive antibodies are present in normal HIV-negative sera." *AIDS Research and Human Retroviruses* 15 (1999): 671–7.
25. Veljković et al., "AIDS epidemic."
26. PB Gilbert, Y-L Chiu, M Allen, et al. "Long-term safety analysis of preventive HIV-1 vaccines evaluated in AIDS vaccine evaluation group: NIAID-sponsored Phase I and II clinical trials." *Vaccine* 211 (2003): 2933–47.
27. Veljković et al., "Does VaxGen hide breakthrough infections?"

CONTROVERSY BREAKS OVER AIDS VACCINE TRIALS

1. D Burton, RC Desrosiers, RW Doms, et al. "A sound rationale needed for phase III HIV-1 vaccine tests." *Science* 303 (16 January 2004): 316.
2. R Belshe, G Franchini, MP Girard, et al. Letters. *Science* 305 (9 July 2004).
3. RC Gallo. Letters. *Science* 305 (9 July 2004).
4. H Urnovitz. "On wasting even more public money on HIV vaccine trials." 7 July 2003. www.redflagsweekly.com/urnovitz/2003_jul07.html
5. JP Roberts. "Are HIV vaccines fighting fire with gasoline?" *The Scientist*, 7 June 2004.
6. F Fleck. "Trials of AIDS vaccines to start in Switzerland and United Kingdom." *British Medical Journal* 326 (3 May 2003): 952. bmj.bmjjournals.com/cgi/content/full/326/7396/952/d
7. "Gp120 vaccines." www.aidsmap.org/en/docs/4406022B-85D7-4A9B-B700-91336CBB6B18.asp
8. "Gp120 vaccines."
9. "Recombinant sub-unit vaccines." www.aidsmap.org/en/docs/C2C88315-792E-4B14-BB37-22F927EE42F2.asp
10. "HIV vaccine trial to commence July 2003 in London and Lausanne." EuroVacc press release, 30 July 2001. www.eurovacc.org/Press/EV01_trial_announcemen.pdf
11. Fleck, op. cit.
12. J Cohen. "AIDS vaccine trial produces disappointment and confusion." *Science* 299 (28 February 2003).
13. Ibid.
14. J Meldrum. "Vaccine research: Back to the drawing board?" aidsmap.com/en/news/046021E2-74CC-42C1-AEE5-5190A6D94E24.asp
15. K Alcorn. "VaxGen announces second phase III trial failure in its AIDSVAX programme." aidsmap.com/en/news/A990B4AA-06B3-4A89-9B23-1629851ECB6C.asp
16. V Suthon, R Archawin, C Chanchai, et al. "Impact of HIV vaccination on laboratory diagnosis: Case reports." *BMC Infectious Diseases* 2 (2002): 19. www.biomedcentral.com/1471-2334/2/19
17. V Veljković, S Muller, H Kohler. "AIDSVAX results: An important open question." *Vaccine* 21 (2003): 3528–9. www.elsevier.com/locate/vaccine
18. V Jirathitikal, P Sooksathan, O Metadilogkul, et al. "V-1 Immunitor: Oral therapeutic AIDS vaccine with prophylactic potential." *Vaccine* 21 (2003): 624–8. www.elsevier.com/locate/vaccine

VACCINATING PEOPLE AGAINST THEIR OWN GENES

1. J Parkin, B Cohen. "An overview of the immune system." *Lancet* 3357 (2001) 1777–89.
2. Medical Encyclopedia, Medline Plus. www.nlm.nih.gov/medlineplus/ency/article/000821.htm#Definition
3. "Cancer and the immune system: The vital connection." OK Dzivenu, J O'Donnell-Tormey. Cancer Research Institute. www.cancerresearch.org/immunology/immuneindex.html
4. L Steinman. "Elaborate interactions between the immune and nervous systems." *Nature Immunology* 5 (2004): 575–81.
5. H Urnovitz, JC Sturge, TD Gottfried, et al. "Urine antibody tests: New insight into the dynamics of HIV-infection." *Clinical Chemistry* 45 (1999): 1602–13.
6. M Clerici, JM Levin, HA Kessler, et al. "HIV-specific T-helper activity in seronegative health care workers exposed to contaminated blood." *Journal of the American Medical Association* 271 (1994): 42–6.
7. LA Pinto, J Sullivan, JA Berzofsky, et al. "ENV-specific cytotoxic T lymphocyte responses in HIV seronegative health care workers occupationally exposed to HIV-contaminated body fluids." *Journal of Clinical Investigation* 96 (1995): 867–76.
8. S Mazzoli, D Trabattoni, S Lo Caputo, et al. "HIV-specific mucosal and cellular immunity in HIV-seronegative partners of HIV-seropositive individuals." *Nature Medicine* 3 (1997): 1250–7.
9. S Rowland-Jones, J Sutton, K Ariyoshi, et al. "HIV-specific cytotoxic T-cells in HIV-exposed but uninfected Gambian women." *Nature Medicine* 1 (1995): 59–64.
10. R Kaul, D Trabattoni, JJ Bwayo, et al. "HIV-1-specific mucosal IgA in a cohort of HIV-1-resistant Kenyan sex workers." *AIDS* 13 (1999): 23–9.
11. AA Kiessling, LM Fitzgerald, D Zhang, et al. "Human immunodeficiency virus in semen arises from a genetically distinct virus reservoir." *AIDS Research and Human Retroviruses* 14 (Suppl 1, 1998): S33–41.
12. M Poss, HL Martin, JK Kreiss, et al. "Diversity in virus populations from genital secretions and peripheral blood from women recently infected with human immunodeficiency virus type 1." *Journal of Virology* 69 (1995): 8118–22.
13. LG Epstein, C Kuiken, BM Blumberg, et al. "HIV-1 V3 domain variation in brain and spleen of children with AIDS: Tissue-specific evolution within host-determined quasispecies." *Virology* 180 (1991): 583–90.
14. AW Artenstein, TC Van Cott, JR Mascola, et al. "Dual infection with human immunodeficiency virus type 1 of distinct envelope subtypes in humans." *Journal of Infectious Diseases* 171 (1995): 805–10.
15. "Infection with more than one HIV strain becoming more common; could complicate vaccine development." *The Body: An AIDS and HIV Information Resource*, 15 July 2003. www.thebody.com/newsroom/2003/jul15_03/multi_hiv.html
16. K Henry. "HIV superinfection 5% in newly infected gay men." The Body: An AIDS and HIV Information Resource, 9 February 2004. www.thebody.com/confs/retro2004/henry1.html

17. N Imami, A Pires, G Hardy, et al. "A balanced type1/type2 response is associated with long-term nonprogressive human immunodeficiency virus type 1 infection." *Journal of Virology* 76 (2002): 9011–23.

18. HB Urnovitz. Written testimony of Dr. Howard B. Urnovitz to U.S. House of Representatives Committee on Government Reform and Oversight, 3 August 1999.

HIV AND LATENT VIRUSES

1. H Urnovitz, JC Sturge, TD Gottfried, et al. "Urine antibody tests: New insight into the dynamics of HIV-infection." *Clinical Chemistry* 45 (1999): 1602–13.

2. HB Urnovitz, JJ Tuite, JM Higashida, et al. "RNAs in the sera of Persian Gulf War veterans have segments homologous to chromosome 22q11.2." *Clinical and Diagnostic Laboratory Immunology* (1999): 330–5.

3. MW Ho, M Hooper. "Dynamic genomics and environmental health." *Science in Society* 19 (2003): 23–5.

4. HB Urnovitz and WH Murphy. "Human endogenous retroviruses: Nature, occurrence, and clinical implications in human disease." *Clinical Microbiology Review* 9 (1996): 72–99.

5. DJ Griffiths. "Endogenous retroviruses in the human genome sequence." *Genome Biology* 2 (no. 6, 2001): reviews 1017.1–1017.5.

6. Y Koga, E Lindstrom, EM Fenyo, et al. "High levels of heterodisperse RNAs accumulate in T cells infected with human immunodeficiency virus and in normal thymocytes." *Proceedings of the National Academy of Sciences U.S.A.* 85 (1988): 4521–5.

7. J Yang, HP Bogerd, S Peng, et al. "An ancient family of human endogenous retroviruses encodes a functional homolog of the HIV-1 Rev protein." *Proceedings of the National Academy of Sciences U.S.A.* 96 (1999): 13404–8.

8. RW Stevens, AL Baltch, RP Smith, et al. "Antibody to human endogenous retrovirus peptide in urine of human immunodeficiency virus type 1-positive patient." *Clinical and Diagnostic Laboratory Immunology* 6 (1999): 783–6.

9. HB Urnovitz. "AIDS: A 'host vs genome' disease with an associated 'virus.'" Statement for the Durban AIDS conference, 4 July 2000. www.chronicillnet.org/AIDS/durban.htm

10. Stevens et al., op. cit.

11. W-M Chu, R Ballard, BW Carpick, et al. "Potential Alu function: Regulation of the activity of double-stranded RNA-activated kinase PKR." *Molecular and Cellular Biology* 18 (1998): 58–68.

12. KL Jang, MKL Collins, DS Latchman. "The human immunodeficiency virus Tat protein increases the transcription of human Alu repeated sequences by increasing the activity of the cellular transcription factor TFIIIC." *Journal of Acquired Immune Deficiency Syndromes* 5 (1992): 1142–7.

13. MW Ho. "Molecular genetic engineers in junk DNA?" *Science in Society* 19 (2003): 28.

14. Urnovitz et al., "RNAs in the sera of Persian Gulf War veterans."

15. Ho and Hooper, op. cit.

16. F Barre-Sinoussi, JC Chermann, F Rey, et al. "Isolation of a T-lymphotropic retrovirus from a patient at risk for acquired immune deficiency syndrome (AIDS)." *Science* 220 (1983): 868–71.

17. GM Shearer. "Natural resistance to parental T-lymphocyte-induced immunosuppression in F1 hybrid mice: Implications for acquired immune deficiency syndrome (AIDS)." *Immunological Reviews* 73 (1983): 115–26.

18. "Chronix Biomedical awarded grant for mad cow disease living test; new blood test only ante mortem diagnostic to address BSE eradication." *Biospace*, 18 April 2005.

19. MW Ho. "Subverting the genetic text." Beyond the Central Dogma series. *Science in Society* 14 (2004): 24.

20. MW Ho. *Living with the Fluid Genome*. London and Penang, Malaysia: ISIS and Third World Network, 2003.

21. N Regush. *The Virus Within*. Toronto: Viking, 2000.

22. P Lusso, RC Gallo. "Human herpesvirus 6 in AIDS." *Immunology Today* 16 (1995): 67–70.

23. LE Fantry, FR Cleghorn. "HHV-6 infection in patients with HIV-1 infection and disease." *AIDS Reader* 9 (1999): 198–221.

24. Ibid.

25. KK Knox, DR Carrigan. "Disseminated active HHV-6 infections in patients with AIDS." *Lancet* 343 (1994): 577.

26. KK Knox, DR Carrigan. "Active human herpesvirus (HHV-6) infection of the central nervous system in patients with AIDS." *Journal of Acquired Immune Deficiency Syndromes and Human Retrovirology* 9 (no. 1, 1995): 69–73.

27. KK Knox, DR Carrigan: "Active HHV-6 infection in the lymph nodes of HIV-infected patients: In vitro evidence that HHV-6 can break HIV latency." *Journal of Acquired Immune Deficiency Syndromes and Human Retrovirology* 11 (1996): 370–8.

28. Regush, op. cit.

THE "PINK PANACEA": AN AIDS VACCINE?

1. "ICHF V-1, the Thai oral therapeutic vaccine for against HIV/AIDS, also scores with diabetes." *International Council for Health Freedom* 7 (nos. 3/4, Winter 2003/Spring 2004): 20–1.

2. V Jirathitikal, P Sooksathan, O Metadilogkul, et al. "V-1 Immunitor: Oral therapeutic AIDS vaccine with prophylactic potential." *Vaccine* 21 (2003): 624–8.

3. V Jirathitikal, O Metadilogkul, AS Bourinbaiar. "Increased body weight and improved quality of life in AIDS patients following V-1 Immunitor administration." *European Journal of Clinical Nutrition* 58 (2004): 110–5.

4. Jirathitikal et al., "V-1 Immunitor."

5. SA Bozette, SH Berry, H Duan, et al. "The care of HIV-infected adults in the United States." *New England Journal of Medicine* 339 (1998): 1897–904.

6. Immunitor Presentation at Keystone Symposium. "HIV Vaccine development: Immunological and Biological Challenges," 29 March–4 April 2003. www.virus-1.com/keystone_symposium.html

7. V Jirathitikal, AS Bourinbaiar. "Low cost anti-HIV compounds: Potential application for AIDS therapy in developing countries." *Current Pharmaceutical Design* 9 (2003): 1419–31.

8. Kenneth Stuart, "Poverty and AIDS," letter to *The Times of London*, 3 December 2003.

9. T Poopat. "10m survive on Bt900 a month." *The Nation*, 20 November 2001.

10. A Treerutkuarkul. "Poverty issue being poorly addressed; better policies needed to tackle problem." *Bangkok Post*, 20 November 2001.

EATING WELL FOR HEALTH

1. PC Calder, S Kew. "The immune system: A target for functional foods?" *British Journal of Nutrition* 88 (Suppl 2, 2002): S165–77.

2. L Amati, D Cirimele, V Pugliese, et al. "Nutrition and immunity: Laboratory and clinical aspects." *Current Pharmaceutical Design* 9 (no. 24, 2003): 1924–31.

3. MT Rivera, AP De Souza, TC Araujo-Jorge, et al. "Trace elements, innate immune response and parasites." *Clinical Chemistry and Laboratory Medicine* 41 (2003): 1020–5.

4. CJ Field, IR Johnson, PD Schley. "Nutrients and their role in host resistance to infection." *Journal of Leukocyte Biology* 71 (2002): 16–32.

5. *McCance and Widdowson's The Composition of Foods*, 5th ed. Royal Society of Chemistry, Ministry of Agriculture, Fisheries and Food, 1992.

6. Field et al., op. cit.

7. Ibid.

8. Ibid.

9. Rivera et al., op. cit.

10. Ibid.

11. Field et al., op. cit.

12. M Tam, S Gomez, M Gonzales-Gross, et al. "Possible roles of magnesium on the immune system." *European Journal of Clinical Nutrition* 57 (2003): 1193–7.

13. Field et al., op. cit.

14. MA Beck. "Selenium and host defence towards viruses." *Proceedings of the Nutrition Society* 58 (1999): 707–11.

15. Amati et al., op. cit.

16. B Lesourd. "Nutrition: A major factor influencing immunity in the elderly." *Journal of Nutrition, Health and Aging* 8 (no. 11, 2004): 28–37.

17. D Krause, AM Mastro, G Handte. "Immune function did not decline with aging in apparently healthy, well-nourished women." *Mechanisms of Ageing and Development* 112 (1999): 43–57.

18. J Fioramonti, V Theodorou, L Bueno. "Probiotics: What are they? What are their effects on gut physiology?" *Best Practice and Research in Clinical Gastroenterology* 17 (2003): 711–24.

19. P Brandtzaeg. "Mucosal immunity: Integration between mother and the breast-fed infant." *Vaccine* 21 (no. 24, 2003): 3382–8.

20. S Sazawal, U Dhingra, A Sarkar, et al. "Efficacy of milk fortified with a probiotic Bifidobacterium lactis (DR-10TM) and prebiotic galacto-oligosaccharides in prevention of morbidity and on nutritional status." *Asia Pacific Journal of Clinical Nutrition* 13 (Suppl, 2004): S28.

21. S Blum, EJ Schiffrin. "Intestinal microflora and homeostasis of the mucosal immune response: Implications for probiotic bacteria?" *Current Issues in Intestinal Microbiology* 4 (2003): 53–60.

22. K Arunachalam, HS Gill, RK Chandra. "Enhancement of natural immune function by dietary consumption of Bifidobacterium lactis (HN019)." *European Journal of Clinical Nutrition* 54 (2000): 263–7.

EATING WELL AGAINST HIV/AIDS

1. WW Fawzi, GI Msamanga, D Spiegelman, et al. "A randomised trial of multi-vitamin supplements and HIV disease progression and mortality." *New England Journal of Medicine* 351 (2004): 23–32.

2. "Guidelines for the use of antiretroviral agents in HIV-1 infected adults and adolescents, April 7, 2005." www.aidsinfo.nih.gov//guidelines/default_db2.asp?id=50

3. B Marston, KM de Cock. "Multivitamins, nutrition and antiretroviral therapy for HIV disease in Africa" (editorial). *New England Journal of Medicine* 351 (2004): 78–80.

4. RD Semba, NM Graham, WT Caiaffa, et al. "Increased mortality associated with vitamin A deficiency during human immunodeficiency virus type 1 infection." *Archives of Internal Medicine* 153 (no. 18, 1993): 2149–54.

5. GO Coodley, MK Coodley, HD Nelson, et al. "Micronutrient concentrations in the HIV wasting syndrome." *AIDS* 7 (no. 12, 1993): 1595–600.

6. JH Skurnick, JD Bogden, H Baker, et al. "Micronutrient profiles in HIV-1-infected heterosexual adults." *Journal of Acquired Immune Deficiency Syndromes and Human Retrovirology* 12 (1996): 75–83.

7. JD Bogden, FW Kemp, S Han, et al. "Status of selected nutrients and progression of human immunodeficiency virus type 1 infection." *American Journal of Clinical Nutrition* 72 (no. 3, 2000): 809–15.

8. MK Baum, G Shor-Posner, Y Lu, et al. "Micronutrients and HIV-1 disease progression." *AIDS* 9 (no. 9, 1995): 1051–6.

9. BA Periquet, NM Jammes, WE Lambert, et al. "Micronutrient levels in HIV-1-infected children." *AIDS* 9 (no. 8, 1995): 887–93.

10. Medical Encyclopaedia, Medline Plus. www.nlm.nih.gov/medlineplus/ency/article/003480.htm

11. P Mastroiacovo, C Ajassa, G Berardelli, et al. "Antioxidant vitamins and immunodeficiency." *International Journal of Vitamin and Nutrition Research* 66 (no. 2, 1996): 141–5.

12. RD Semba, PG Miotti, JD Chiphangwi, et al. "Infant mortality and maternal vitamin A deficiency during human immunodeficiency virus infection." *Clinical Infectious Disease* 21 (no. 4, 1995): 966–72.

13. D Rakower, TA Galvin. "Nourishing the HIV-infected adult." *Holistic Nursing Practice* 3 (no. 4, 1989): 26–37.
14. L Patrick. "Nutrients and HIV, part three. N-acetylcysteine, alpha-lipoic acid, L-glutamine, and L-carnitine." *Alternative Medicine Review* 5 (no. 4, 2000): 290–305.
15. S Harakeh, Jariwalla RJ. "Ascorbate effect on cytokine stimulation of HIV production." *Nutrition* 1995, 11 (Suppl 5, 1995): 684–7.
16. S Harakeh, RJ Jariwalla. "Ascorbate effect on cytokine stimulation of HIV production." *Nutrition* 11 (Suppl 5, 1995): 684–7.
17. CI Rivas, JC Vera, VH Guaiquil. "Effects of trace metal compounds on HIV-1 reverse transcriptase: An in vitro study." *Biological Trace Element Research* 68 (no. 2, 1999): 107–19.
18. WW Fawzi, GI Msamanga, D Spiegelman, et al. "Randomised trial of effects of vitamin supplements on pregnancy outcomes and T cell counts in HIV-1-infected women in Tanzania." *Lancet* 351 (16 May 1998): 1477–82.
19. E Villamor, G Msamanga, D Spiegelman, et al. "Effect of multivitamin and vitamin A supplements on weight gain during pregnancy among HIV-1-infected women." *American Journal of Clinical Nutrition* 76 (no. 5, 2002): 1082–90.
20. AM Tang, NM Graham, AJ Saah. "Effects of micronutrient intake on survival in human immunodeficiency virus type 1 infection." *American Journal of Epidemiology* 143 (no. 12, 1996): 1244–56.
21. DA De Luis, P Bachiller, R Aller, et al. "Relation among micronutrient intakes with CD4 count in HIV infected patients." *Nutricion Hospitalaria* 17 (no. 6, 2002): 285–9.

SELENIUM CONQUERS AIDS

1. HD Foster. "AIDS and the 'selenium-CD4 T cell tailspin': The geography of a pandemic." *Townsend Letter from Doctors and Patients*, December 2000.
2. MK Baum, G Shor-Posner, S Lai, et al. "High risk of HIV related mortality is associated with selenium deficiency." *Journal of Acquired Immune Deficiency Syndromes and Human Retrovirology* 15 (no. 5, 1997): 370–4.
3. UNAIDS/WHO. "Epidemiological fact sheet on HIV/AIDS and sexually transmitted infections: Senegal." 2000 Update (revised).
4. GM Howe. "International variations in cancer incidence and mortality," in *Global Geocancerology: A World Geography of Human Cancers*. New York: Churchill Livingston, 1986, 3–42.
5. DG Janelle, B Warf, K Hansen, eds. *Worldminds: Geographical Perspectives on 100 Problems*. Dordrecht, Netherlands: Kluwar Academic Publishers, 2004, 69–73.
6. Foster, "AIDS and the 'selenuim-CD4 T cell tailspin.'"
7. HD Foster. "How HIV-1 causes AIDS: Implications for prevention and treatment." *Medical Hypotheses* 62 (no. 4, 2004): 549–53.
8. R Giraldo. "Southern African Development Community (SADC) Meeting on Nutrition and HIV/AIDS." Johannesburg, South Africa, 28–29 November 2002. www.robertogiraldo.com/eng/papers/ReportOfSADCMeeting.html
9. Baum et al., op. cit.

10. B McIntyre. "HIV/AIDS and complementary therapies."
www.positivelypositive.ca/articles/therapies.html
11. J Kirkham, J Whitehead. "Some immune stimulating treatments and the scientific basis for them." www.altheal.org/treatments/oxidative.htm
12. Foster, "How HIV-1 causes AIDS."
13. WH Fuller. "Movement of selected metals, asbestos, and cyanide in soil: Applications to waste disposal problem." EPA-6000/2-77020-Cincinnati: Solid and Hazardous Waste Research Division. EPA, 1977.
14. J Last. "Potential health effects of global change." *Delta* 2 (no. 2, 1991): 1–6.
15. GF Combs Jr, ML Scott. "Polychlorinated biphenyl-stimulated selenium deficiency in the chick." *Poultry Science* 54 (no. 4, 1975): 1152–8.
16. P Micke, KM Beeh, JF Schlaak, et al. "Oral supplementation with whey proteins increase plasma glutathione levels of HIV infected patients." *European Journal of Clinical Investigation* 31 (no. 2, February 2001): 171–8.
17. JP Allard, E Aghdassi, J Chau, et al. "Effects of vitamin E and C supplementation on oxidative stress and viral load in HIV–infected subjects." *AIDS* 12 (no. 13, September 10, 1998): 1653–9.
18. RS Beach, E Mantero-Atienza, G Shor-Posner, et al. "Specific nutrient abnormalities in asymptomatic HIV-1 infection." *AIDS* 6 (no. 7, 1992): 701–8.
19. S Burcher. "European Directive Against Vitamins and Minerals." *Science in Society* 20 (Autumn/Winter 2003): 40–1.

PROBIOTICS FOR LIFE AFTER HIV/AIDS

1. Sandor Ellix Katz. Wild Fermentation. www.wildfermentation.com
2. R Wood. Healing with food; food as medicine; fermented foods strengthen immune system. www.rwood.com/index.htm
3. R Giraldo. "An effective prevention for AIDS." June 2000. www.virusmyth.net/aids/data/rgprevention.htm
4. M Konlee. "Th 1 probiotics are finally here." *Positive Health News*, Spring 2000. www.keephopealive.org/report20.html
5. M Konlee. "The colon and the critical pH factor: Why an acidic colon is of immeasurable value to persons immune compromised." *Positive Health News*, Fall 1999. www.keephopealive.org/report19.html
6. M Konlee. "A self-help guide for the immune compromised." *Positive Health News*, Spring 2001. www.keephopealive.org/report22.html
7. M Konlee. "The many benefits of friendly intestinal flora." *Positive Health News*, Spring 2000. www.keephopealive.org/report20.html
8. A Korotzer. "The gut reaction to HIV." *Searchlight*, Winter 1999. www.aidsresearch.org/winter2a.html
9. G Pantaleo, C Graziosi, JF Demarest, et al. "HIV infection is active and progressive in lymphoid tissue during the clinically latent stage of disease" (abstract). *Nature* 362 (1993): 355–8.
10. M Konlee. "A consumer's guide to immune restoration: The search for Th1." *Positive Health News*, Spring 1999. www.keephopealive.org/report18.html

11. RJ Darga. "Cytokines and cellular immunity." *Positive Health News*, June 1997. www.keephopealive.org/report14.html

12. Darga, op. cit.

13. Konlee, "Consumer's guide."

14. IM Bovee-Oudenhoven, ML Wissink, JT Wouters, et al. "Dietary calcium phosphate stimulates intestinal Lactobacilli and decreases the severity of a Salmonella infection in rats." *Journal of Nutrition* 129 (1999): 607–12.

15. M Konlee. "Acidophilus and the calcium factor." *Positive Health News*, Spring 2000. www.keephopealive.org/report20.html

HERBS FOR IMMUNITY

1. "The anatomy of the immune system." www.micro.msb.le.ac.uk/mbchb/2b.html

2. R Gair. "The good, the bad and the toxic." *Positive Living*, September/October 2001, 18–9.

3. IB Stehlin, "An FDA guide to choosing medical treatments." *FDA Consumer*, June 1995. www.fda.gov/oashi/aids/fdaguide.html

4. D Hoffman. *Holistic Herbal*. London: HarperCollins, 2002, 129–30.

5. MW Ho. *Living with the Fluid Genome*. London and Penang, Malaysia: ISIS and Third World Network, 2003.

6. S Burcher, MW Ho. "Global strategy for traditional medicine." *Science in Society* 16 (2002): 23–5.

7. Y Ma, Z Tian, H Kuang, et al. "Studies of the constituents of Astragalus membrananeous." *Chemical Pharmacological Bulletin* 45 (1997): 359–61.

8. K Kemper, R Small. "Astragalus (*Astragalus membranaceous*)." Longwood Herbal Taskforce, Center for Holistic Paediatric Education and Research, rev. 3 September 1999. www.mcphs.edu/MCPHSWeb/herbal/astragalus/astragalus.cis.PDF

9. N El-Sebakhy, A Asaad, R Abdullah, et al. "Antimicrobial isoflavan from Astragalus species." *Phytochemistry* 36 (1994): 1387–9.

10. W Goux, S Boyd, C Tone, et al. "Effects of glyconutritional on oxidative stress on human subject: A pilot study." *Glycoscience and Nutrition* 2 (8 June 2001): 12.

11. D Chu, J Lin, W Wong. "The in vitro potential of LAK cell cytotoxicity in cancer and AIDS patients induced by F3, a fractionated extract of astragalus membranaceous." *Chinese Journal of Oncology* 16 (1994): 167–71.

12. Y Yoshida, M Wang, J Liu, et al. "Immonomodulating activity of Chinese medical herbs and Oldenlandia diffusia in particular." *International Journal of Immunopharmacology* 19 (1997): 359–70.

13. UNICEF. "Epidemiological fact sheets on HIV/AIDS and sexually transmitted infections." hivinsite.ucsf.edu/pdf/UNAIDS/China_en.pdf

14. L Jagen. "Asia warned of AIDS epidemic." BBC Asia Pacific Online, 5 October 2001.

15. TK Yun, SY Choi. "Preventative effect of ginseng intake against various human cancers: A case controlled study on 1987 pairs." *Cancer Epidemiology, Biomarkers, and Prevention* (no. 4, 4 June 1995): 401–8.

16. G Pieralisi, P Ripari, L Vecchiet. "Effects of standardized ginseng extracts combined with dimethyaminoethenal bitartrate, vitamins, minerals and trace elements on physical performance during exercise." *Clinical Therapy* 13 (no. 3, May–June 1991): 373–82.

17. AW Ziemna, J Chmura, Kaciuba-Uscilko, et al. "Ginseng treatment improves psychomotor performance at rest and during graded exercise in young athletes." *International Journal of Sports Nutrition* 4 (9 December 1999): 371–7.

18. F Scaglione, F Ferrara, S Dugnani, et al. "Immunomodulatory effects of two extracts of Panax Ginseng C Meyer." *Drugs Under Experimental and Clinical Research* 16 (no. 10, 1990): 337–42.

19. M Mizuno, J Yamada, H Terai, et al. "Differences in immunomodulating effects between wild and cultured Panax ginseng." *Biochemical and Biophysical Research Communications* 3 (1994): 1672–8.

20. JS Montaner, J Gill, J Singer, et al. "Double blind placebo-controlled pilot trial of acemannan in advanced human immunodeficiency virus disease." *Journal of Acquired Immune Deficiency Syndromes and Human Retrovirology* 12 (no. 2, 1 June 1996): 153–7.

21. T Pulse. "A study of 29 AIDS patients." *Journal of Advancement in Medicine* 3 (Winter 1990): 4.

22. Texas A&M University. "Substance boosts therapeutic effects of AZT." *AIDS Weekly* 119 (no. 2, 5 August 1991): 2.

23. WV Cruess, CL Alsberg. "The bitter glucoside of the olive." *Journal of American Chemotherapy Society* 56 (1934): 2115–7.

24. HE Renis. "In vitro antiviral activity of calcium elenolate." *Antimicrobial Agents and Chemotherapy* (1970): 167–72.

25. J James. "Naltrexone safety note: Dosage error." www.aids.org/atn/a-052-04.html

26. N Ikegami, et al. "Clinical evaluation of glycyrrhizin on HIV infection in asymptomatic haemophiliac patients in Japan." V International Conference on AIDS (abstract WBP 298), June 1989.

27. K Mori, H Sakai, S Suzuki, et al. "Effects of glycyrrhizin in haemophiliac patients with HIV infection." *Tohoku Journal of Experimental Medicine* 158 (1989): 25–35.

28. M Konlee. "A case report: Treating HIV with neem and guaifenesin." *Journal of Immunity* 1 (October–December 2003): 3.

29. Y Yamada, K Azuma. "Evaluation of the in vitro antifungal activity of allicin." *Antimicrobial Agents and Chemotherapy* 4 (11 April 1977): 743–9.

30. TH Abdullah, DV Kirkpatrick, J Carter. "Enhancement of natural killer cell activity in AIDS with garlic." *Deutsche Zeitschrift Onkologie* 21 (1989): 52–3.

31. O Kandil, T Abdullah, AM Tabuni, et al. "Potential role of Allium sativuum in natural cytotoxicity." *Archives of AIDS Research* 1 (1998): 230–1.

32. HD Reuter, HP Koch, LD Lawson. "Therapeutic effects and application of garlic and its preparations," in *Garlic: The Science and Therapeutic Application of Allium sativuum L and Related Species.* Williams & Wilkins, 1996, 135–212.

33. H Neychev, V Dimoy, V Vulveva, et al. "Immunomodulatory action of propolis. II. Effect of water soluable fraction on influenza infection in mice." *Acta Microbial Bulgaria* 23 (1988): 58–62.

34. RO Orsi, SRC Funari, AMVC Soares, et al. "Immunomodulatory action of propolis on macrophage activation." *Journal of Venomous Animals and Toxins Including Tropical Diseases* 6 (no. 2, 2000): 205–19.

35. D Morrison. "Propolis: An ancient remedy may fight AIDS." University of Minnesota News, 24 May 2004. www1.umn.edu/umnnews/Feature_Stories/ Propolis_an_ancient_remedy_may_fight_AIDS.html

36. K Flora, M Hahn, H Rosen, et al. *American Journal of Gastroenterology* 198 (no. 2, February 1993): 139–43.

TRADITIONAL MEDICINE IN THE FIGHT AGAINST AIDS

1. D Hoffman. *Holistic Herbal*. London: Harper Collins, 2002.

2. "WHO Traditional Medicine Strategy 2002–2005." Geneva: World Health Organization, 2002. www.who.int/medicines/library/trm/trm_strat_eng.pdf3

3. S Burcher, MW Ho. "Global strategy for traditional medicine." *Science in Society* 16 (2002): 23.

4. P Goldblatt, JC Manning. *Cape Plants: A Conspectus of the Cape Flora of South Africa*. Pretoria, SA, and St. Louis, Mo.: National Botanical Institute, Botanical Garden Press, 2000.

5. AD Smith. "Race to stop drug firms patenting African plant that helps AIDS victims." *The Independent*, 30 November 2001. news.independent.co.uk/low_res/ story.jsp?story=107518&host=3&dir=69

6. A Hutchings. "A personal and scientifically based perspective on indigenous herbal medicines in the treatment of HIV and AIDS: A clinic experience." Paper presented to the MRC KZN AIDS Forum, 29 October 2002, University of Zululand.

7. Smith, op. cit.

8. Hutchings, op. cit.

9. Smith, op. cit.

10. N Gericke. "Sutherlandia and AIDS patients: An update." *Australian Journal of Medical Herbalism* 13 (no. 1, March 2003).

11. CA Smith. "Common names of South African plants." Botantical survey memoir no. 35. Pretoria, SA: Government printer, 1996.

12. PA Crooks, GA Rosenthal. "Use of L-canavanine as a chemotherapeutic agent for the treatment of pancreatic cancer." United States patent 5,552,440, filed 5 December 1994.

13. "Herbal treatment for AIDS." *Daily Dispatch* (South Africa), 15 March 2001. www.dispatch.co.za/2001/03/15/southafrica/BAIDS.HTM

14. "*Sutherlandia* and HIV/AIDS." www.sutherlandia.org/aids.html

15. JV Seier, M Mdhluli, MA Dhansay, et al. "A toxicity study of *Sutherlandia* leaf powder (*Sutherlandia mycrophylla*) consumption." Medical Research Council of South Africa and National Research Foundation. www.sahealthinfo.org/ traditionalmeds/sutherlandia.pdf

16. N Walters. "Corporate reports: Indigenous knowledge systems (health)." Medical Research Council of South Africa. www.mrc.ac.za/annualreport/culture.htm

17. Stuart Thomson rebuts Dr. Mohapeloa. "*Sutherlandia*: Poison as a panacea." *Druginfo*, August 2002. www.gaiaresearch.co.za/sutherlandia3.html
18. F Haffajee. "Home grown healing." *New Internationalist* 349 (September 2002).
19. J Tai, S Cheung S, E Chan, et al. "In vitro culture studies of *Sutherlandia frutescens* on human tumour cell lines." *Journal of Ethnopharmacology* 93 (2004): 9–19.
20. C Smith, KH Myburgh. "Treatment of *Sutherlandia frutesecens ssp. microphylla* alters the corticosterone response to chronic intermittent immobilization stress in rats." *South African Journal of Science* (2004): 229–232.
21. AC Fernandes, AD Cromarty, C Albrecht, et al. "The antioxidant potential of *Sutherlandia frutescens*." *Journal of Ethnopharmacology* 95 (no. 1, November 2004): 1–5.
22. S Burcher. "Rolling back malaria." *Science in Society* 13/14 (2002): 29.
23. C Dempster. "Medicinal plant 'fights' AIDS." BBC News, 30 November 2001. news.bbc.co.uk/1/hi/world/africa/1683259.stm
24. G Vince. "Clinical trial for herbal AIDS treatment." *New Scientist*, 30 November 2001. www.newscientist.com/article.ns?id=dn1632

HYPERICUM VERSUS HIV/AIDS

1. Anonymous. "*Hypericum*." *Alternative Medicine Review* 4 (no. 3, 1999).
2. D Meruelo, G Lavie, D Lavie. "Therapeutic agents with dramatic antiviral activity and little toxicity at effective doses: Aromatic polycyclic diones Hypericum and pseudohypericin." *Proceedings of the National Academy of Sciences* 85 (no. 14, July 1988): 5230–4.
3. S Degar, AM Prince, D Pascual, et al. "Inactivation of the human immunodeficiency virus by hypericin: Evidence for phytochemical alterations of P24 and a block in uncoating AIDS." *AIDS Research and Human Retroviruses* 8 (1992): 1929–36.
4. A Steinbeck-Klose, et al. "Successful long-term treatment over 40 months of HIV positive patients with intravenous hypericin." Ninth International Conference on AIDS, Berlin, 1993, abstract B26–2012.
5. WC Cooper, J James. "An observational study of the safety and efficacy of hypericin in HIV+ subjects." International Conference on AIDS, 20–23 June 1990, 6 (no. 2): 369, abstract 2063.
6. JB Hudson, I Lopez-Bazzocchi. "Antiviral activity of photoactive plant pigment hypericin." *Photochemistry and Photobiology* 54 (no. 1, July 1991): 95–8.
7. J Lenard, A Rabson, R Vanderoef. "Photodynamic inactivation of infectivity of human immunodeficiency virus and other enveloped viruses using hypericin and rose bengal: Inhibition of fusion and syncytia formation." *Proceedings of the National Academy of Sciences U.S.A.* 90 (no. 1, 1993): 158–62.
8. JB Hudson, L Harris, GHN Towers. "The importance of light in the anti-HIV effect of hypericin." *Antiviral Research* 20 (no. 2, 1993): 173–8.
9. GA Kraus, D Pratt, J Tossberg, et al. "Antiretroviral activity of synthetic hypericin and related analogs." *Biochemical and Biophysical Research Communications* 172 (no. 1, 1990): 149–53.

10. G Lavie, F Valentine, D Lavie, et al. "Studies of the mechanisms of action of the antiretroviral agents hypericin and pseudohypericin." *Proceedings of the National Academy of Sciences U.S.A.* 85 (no. 15, 1988): 5963–7.

11. J Tang, JM Colaccino, SH Larsen, et al. "Virucidal activity of hypericin against enveloped and non-enveloped DNA and RNA viruses." *Antiviral Research* 13 (1990): 313–25.

12. I Takahashi, S Nakanishi, E Kobayashi, et al. "Hypericin and pseudohypericin specifically inhibit protease kinase C: Possible relation to the antiviral activity." *Research Communications* 165 (no. 3, 29 December 1989): 1207–12.

13. AG Panossian, E Gabrielian, V Manvelian, et al. "Immunosuppressive effects of hypericin on stimulated human leukocytes: Inhibition of the arachidonic acid release, leukotriene B4 and interleukin-1 alpha production, and activation of nitric oxide formation." *Phytomedicine* 3 (no. 1, 1996): 19–28.

14. G Lavie, Y Mazur, D Lavie, et al. "Hypericin as an inactivator of infectious viruses in blood components." *Transfusion* 35 (no. 5, 1995): 392–400.

15. P Pitisuttithum, S Migasena, P Suntharasamai, et al. "Hypericin: Safety and antiretroviral activity in Thai HIV positive volunteers." *International Conference on AIDS*, 7–12 July 1996, 11 (no. 1): 285, abstract Tu-B-2121.

16. CP Seigers, S Biel, KP Wilhelm. Zur Frage der Phototoxiztat von Hypericum. *Nervenheilkunde* 12 (1993): 320–2.

17. J Brakmoller, T Reum, S Baver, et al. "Hypericin and pseudohypericin pharma-cokinetics and effects on photosensitivity in humans." *Pharmacological Psychiatry* 30 (1997): S94–S101.

18. R Gulick, V McAuliffe, J Holden-Wiltse, et al. "Phase one studies of hypericin, the active compound in St. John's wort, as an antiretroviral agent in HIV infected adults: AIDS clinical trials Group Protocols 150 and 258." *Annals of Internal Medicine* 130 (March 1999): 510–4.

19. EU Vorbach, KH Arnoldt, WD Hubner. "Efficacy and tolerability of St. John's wort extract LI 160 versus imipramine in patients with severe depressive episodes according to ICD-10." *Pharmacopsychiatry* 30 (no. 2, September 1997): S81–5.

20. SN Okpanyi, H Lidzba, BC Scholl, et al. "Genotoxicity of a standardized hypericum extract." *Arzneimittelforschung* 40 (no. 8, August 1990): 851–5.

21. OS Araya and EJH Ford. "An investigation of the type of photosensitization caused by the ingestion of St. John's wort (*Hypericum perforatum*) by calves." *Journal of Comparative Pathology* 91 (no. 1, 1981): 135–141.

22. Seigers et al., op cit.

THERAPEUTIC MUSHROOMS

1. G Chihara, J Hamuro, Y Maeda, et al. "Antitumor and metastasis inhibitory activities of lentinan as an immunomodulator." *Cancer Detection and Prevention* 1 (1987): 423–43.

2. G Chihara, J Hamuro, Y Maeda, et al. "Fractionation and purification of the polysaccharides with marked antitumor activity, especially lentinan, from

Lentinus edodes (Berk.) Sing. (an edible mushroom)." *Cancer Research* 30 (1970): 2776–81.

3. www.cancer.org/docroot/ETO/content/ETO_5_3X_Coriolous_ Versicolor.asp?sitearea=ETO

4. K Harwood, C Pickett. *A Cancer Patient's Guide to Complementary and Alternative Medicine*, ed. 2. Durham, NC, and Santa Barbara, CA: Duke University Medical Center and Cancer Center of Santa Barbara, 2000, 71.

5. M Torisu, Y Jayashi, T Ishimitsu, et al. "Significant prolongation of disease-free period gained by oral polysaccharide K (PSK) administration after curative surgical operation of colorectal cancer." *Cancer* 31 (1990): 261–8.

6. H Nakatazato, A Koike, S Saji, et al. "Efficacy of immunochemotherapy as adjuvant treatment after curative resection of gastric cancer: Study group of immunochemotherapy with PSK for gastric cancer." *Lancet* 343 (1994): 1122–6.

7. J Munro. "Pioneering work at Breakspear Hospital on Coriolus supplementation for CFIDS/ME patients." *Mycology News* 1 (December 2000): 4.

8. J Munro. "Cytokine TH1 response vs. cytokine TH2 immune response." *Mycology News* 1 (July 2001): 5.

9. M Pfeiffer. "The clinical use of Coriolus versicolor supplementation in HIV+ patients and its impact on CD4 count and viral load." *Mycology News* 1 (July 2001): 5.

10. H Nanba, AM Hamaguchi, H Kuroda. "The chemical structure of an anti-tumour polysaccharide in fruit bodies of Grifola frondosa (maitake)." *Chemical Pharmalogical Bulletin* 35 (no. 3, March 1987): 1172–8.

11. H Nanba. "Maitake D-fraction: Healing and preventative potential for cancer." www.orthomed.org/links/papers/namba.htm

12. M Gordon, B Bihari, E Goosby, et al. "A placebo-controlled trial of the immune modulator lentinan on HIV-positive patients: A phase I/II trial." *Journal of Medicine* 29 (nos. 5–6, 1998): 305–30.

13. M Gordon et al. "A phase II controlled study of a combination of the immune modulator, lentinan, with didanosine (ddI) in HIV patients with CD4 cells of 200-500/mm^3." *Journal of Medicine* 26 (nos. 5–6, 1995): 193–207.

14. S Sarkar, J Koga, RJ Whitley, et al. "Antiviral effect of the extract of culture medium of Lentinus edodes mycelia on the replication of herpes simplex virus type 1." *Antiviral Research* (no. 4, April 1993): 293–303.

15. P C Calder. "Immunonutrition may have beneficial effects in surgical patients." *British Medical Journal* 327 (19 July 2003): 117–8.

16. www.seedsofhealth.co.uk/fermenting/kombucha.shtml

AIDS THERAPY FROM CHEAP GENERICS

1. AS Bourinbaiar, V Jirathitikal. "Low-cost anti-HIV compounds: Potential application for AIDS therapy in developing countries." *Current Pharmaceutical Design* 9 (2003): 1419–31.

2. JP Aymard, B Aymard, P Netter, et al. "Haematological adverse effects of histamine H2-receptor antagonists." *Medical Toxicology and Adverse Drug Experience* 3 (1988): 430–48.

3. NH Brockmeyer, E Kreuzfelder, L Mertins, et al. "Immunomodulatory properties of cimetidine in ARC patients." *Clinical Immunology and Immunopathology* 48 (1988): 50–60.

4. E Kouassi, G Caille, L Lery, et al. "Novel assay and pharmacokinetics of levamisole and p-hydroxylevamisole in human plasma and urine." *Biopharmaceutics and Drug Disposition* 7 (1986): 71–89.

5. Bourinbaiar and Jirathitikal, op. cit.

6. AS Bourinbaiar, S Lee-Huang. "The non-steroidal anti-inflammatory drug, indomethacin, as an inhibitor of HIV replication." *FEBS Letters* 360 (1995): 85–8.

7. Ibid.

8. MA Otten-Kuipers, FF Franssen, H Nieuwenhuijs, et al. "Effect of tryptophan-N-formylated gramicidin on growth of Plasmodium berghei in mice." *Antimicrobial Agents and Chemotherapy* 41 (1997): 1778–82.

9. C Gumila, ML Ancelin, AM Delort. "Characterization of the potent in vitro and in vivo antimalarial activities of ionophore compounds." *Antimicrobial Agents and Chemotherapy* 41 (1997): 523–9.

10. AS Bourinbaiar, CF Coleman. "The effect of gramicidin, a topical contraceptive and antimicrobial agent with anti-HIV activity, against herpes simplex viruses type 1 and 2 in vitro." *Archives of Virology* 142 (1997): 2225–35.

11. AS Bourinbaiar, K Krasinski, W Borkowsky. "Anti-HIV effect of gramicidin in vitro: Potential for spermicide use." *Life Sciences* 54 (1994): PL5–9.

12. AS Bourinbaiar, S Lee-Huang. "Comparative in vitro study of contraceptive agents with anti-HIV activity: Gramicidin, nonoxynol-9, and gossypol." *Contraception* 49 (1994): 131–7.

EXERCISE VERSUS AIDS

1. V Veljković, R Metlaš, H Kohler, et al. "AIDS epidemic at the beginning of the third millennium: Time for a new AIDS vaccine strategy." *Vaccine* 19 (2001): 1855–62.

2. H Kohler, S Muller, V Veljković. "No hope for an AIDS vaccine soon." *AIDScience* 2 (2002): 5–6.

3. V Veljković, E Johnson, R Metlaš. "Molecular basis of the inefficacy and possible harmful effects of AIDS vaccine candidates based on HIV-1 envelope glycoprotein gp120." *Vaccine* 15 (1997): 437–8.

4. V Veljković, S Muller, H Kohler. "Does VaxGen hide the breakthrough infections?" *Lancet* 361 (2003): 1743–4.

5. V Veljković, S Muller, H Kohler. "AIDSVAX results: An important open question." *Vaccine* 21 (2003): 3528–9.

6. AR Neurath, N Strick, P Taylor. "Search for epitope-specific antibody responses to the HIV-1 envelope glycoprotein signifying resistance to disease development." *AIDS Research and Human Retroviruses* 6 (1990): 1183–92.

7. V Veljković, R Metlaš, DJ Jevtovic, et al. "The role of passive immunization in HIV-positive patients: A case report." *Chest* 120 (2001): 662–6.

8. V Veljković, R Metlaš, J Raspopovic, et al. "Spectral and sequence similarity between VIP and the second conserved region of HIV envelope glycoprotein

gp120: Possible consequences on prevention and therapy of AIDS." *Biochemical and Biophysical Research Commununications* 189 (1992): 705–10.

9. V Veljković, R Metlaš, D Vojvodic. "Natural autoantibodies cross-react with a peptide derived from the second conserved region of HIV-1 envelope glycoprotein gp120." *Biochemical and Biophysical Research Communications* 196 (1993): 1019–24.

10. Veljković et al., "Natural antibodies cross-react."

11. S Paul, SI Said. "Human autoantibody to vasoactive intestinal peptide: Increased incidence in muscular exercise." *Life Sciences* 43 (1988): 1079–84.

12. V Veljković, R Metlaš. "HIV and idiotypic T-cell regulation: Another view." *Immunology Today* 15 (1992): 39–40.

13. R Metlaš, D Trajkovic, T Srdic, et al. "Human immunodeficency virus V3 peptide-reactive antibodies are present in normal HIV-negative sera." *AIDS Research and Human Retroviruses* 15 (1999): 671–7.

14. R Metlaš, D Trajkovic, T Srdic, et al. "Anti-V3 and anti-IgG antibodies of healthy individuals share complementarity structures." *Journal of Acquired Immune Deficiency Syndromes* 21 (1999): 266–70.

15. R Metlaš, V Veljković. "Does HIV-1 gp120 manipulate human immune network?" *Vaccine* 13 (1995): 355–9.

16. Veljković et al., "AIDS epidemic."

17. Veljković et al., "Does VaxGen hide the breakthrough infections?"

18. Veljković et al., "AIDSVAX results."

19. M McElrath, L Corey, PD Greenberg, et al. "Human immunodeficiency virus type 1 infection despite prior immunization with a recombinant envelope vaccine regimen." *Proceedings of the National Academy of Sciences U.S.A.* 93 (1996): 3972–6.

20. CP Locher, RM Grant, EA Collisson, et al. "Antibody and cellular immune responses in breakthrough infection subjects after HIV type 1 glycoprotein 120 vaccination." *AIDS Research and Human Retroviruses* 71 (1999): 1685–9.

21. Neurath et al., op. cit.

22. JA Bradac, BJ Mathieson. "An epitope map of immunity to HIVHIV-1: A roadmap for vaccine development." Division of AIDS, National Institute of Allergy and Infectious Diseases, National Institutes of Health, NIAID, 1991.

23. V Veljković, E Johnson, R Metlaš. "Analogy of HIV-1 to oncogenic viruses: Possible implications for the pathogenesis of AIDS." *Cancer Journal* 8 (1995): 308–12.

24. Veljković et al., "Spectral and sequence similarity."

25. Veljković et al., "Natural autoantibodies cross-react."

26. M Peruzzi, C Azzari, ME Rossi, et al. "Inhibition of natural killer cell cytotoxicity and interferon gamma production by the envelope protein of HIV and prevention by vasoactive intestinal peptide." *AIDS Research and Human Retroviruses* 16 (2000): 1067–74.

27. V Veljković, R Metlaš. "Identification of nanopeptide from HTLV3, LAV and ARV-2 envelope gp120 determining binding to T4 cell surface protein." *Cancer Biochemistry and Biophysics* 10 (1988): 191–206.

28. V Veljković et al (unpublished).

29. Neurath et al., op. cit.

30. Paul and Said, op. cit.

31. L Woie, B Kaada, PK Opstad. "Increase in plasma vasoactive intesinal polypeptide (VIP) in muscular exercise in humans." *General Pharmacology* 17 (1986): 321–9.

32. DP MacLaren. "Human gastrin and vasoactive intestinal polypeptide responses to endurance running in relation to training status and fluid ingested." *Clinical Science* 89 (1995): 137–46.

33. J Johnson, G Anders, H Blanton, et al. "Exercise dysfunction in patients seropositive for the human immunodeficiency virus-1." *American Review of Respiratory Diseases* 141 (1990): 618–25.

34. WW Stringer. "HIV and aerobic exercise: Current recommendations." *Sports Medicine* 28 (1999): 387–97.

35. PE Olson, MR Wallace, M Carl. "CD4+ correlates of weight training in HIV-seropositive outpatients." *National Conference on Human Retroviruses and Related Information* 2 (1995): 155.

36. PE Olson, H Elrick, GR Cohan, et al. "Non-detectable quantitative HIV PCR in a long-term survivor triathlete" (abstract no. We.C.3472). *International Conference on AIDS* 11 (1996): 140.

37. A LaPerriere, N Klimas, MA Fletcher, et al. "Change in CD4+ cell enumeration following aerobic exercise training in HIV-1 disease: Possible mechanisms and practical applications." *International Journal of Sports Medicine* 18 (Suppl 1, 1997): S56–S63.

38. T Mustafa, FS Sy, CA Macera, et al. "Association between exercise and HIV disease progression in a cohort of homosexual men." *Annals of Epidemiology* 9 (1999): 127–39.

39. BA Smith, J Neidig, J Nickel, et al. "Effects of aerobic and resistive exercise on symptoms, immune status, and viral load in HIV+ men and women" (abstract no. Mo.B.304). *International Conference on AIDS* 11 (1996): 23.

40. BA Smith, J Neidig, J Nickel, et al. "Effects of aerobic and resistive exercise training on body composition, immune markers, and viral load in HIV+ adults with CD4+ counts 200-499/mm3" (abstract no. 42328). *International Conference on AIDS* 12 (1998): 839.

41. RJ Shephard. "Exercise, immune function and HIV infection." *Journal of Sports Medicine and Physical Fitness* 38 (1998): 101–7.

42. RD MacArthur, SD Levine, TJ Berk. "Supervised exercise training improves cardiopulmonary fitness in HIV-infected persons." *Medicine and Science in Sports and Exercise* 25 (1993): 684–97.

43. FM Perna, A LaPerriere, NG Klimas, et al. "Cardiopulmonary and CD4 changes in response to exercise training in early symptomatic HIV infection." *Medicine and Science in Sports and Exercise* 31 (1999): 973–82.

44. G Pothoff, K Wasserman, H Ostmann. "Impairment of exercise capacity in various groups of HIV-infected patients." *Respiration* 61 (1994): 80–5.

45. LW Rigsby, RK Dishman, AW Jackson, et al. "Effects of exercise training on men seropositive for the human immunodeficiency virus-1." *Medicine and Science in Sports and Exercise* 24 (1992): 6–14.

46. WW Stringer, M Berezovskaya, WA O'Brien, et al. "The effect of exercise training on aerobic fitness, immune indices, and quality of life in HIV+ patients." *Medicine and Science in Sports and Exercise* 30 (1998): 11–17.

47. L Terry, E Sprinz, JP Ribeiro. "Moderate and high intensity exercise training in HIV-1 seropositive individuals: A randomized trial." *International Journal of Sports Medicine* 20 (1999): 142–8.

48. Stringer, op. cit.

49. Olson et al., "CD4+ correlates of weight training."

50. Olson et al., "Non-detectable quantitative HIV PCR."

51. LaPerriere et al., op. cit.

52. Mustafa et al., op. cit.

53. Smith et al., "Effects of aerobic and resistive exercise," 1996.

54. Smith et al., "Effects of aerobic and resistive exercise," 1998.

55. Shephard, op. cit.

THE WAY AHEAD

1. D Rasnick. "An abuse of surrogate markers for AIDS." Rapid Responses to News Extra: D Spurgeon, "Canadian aboriginals in Vancouver face AIDS epidemic." *British Medical Journal* 326 (2003), 126e.

2. RS Hawa. "Africa and the virus of underdevelopment," in *AIDS: In Search of a Social Solution*. Penang, Malaysia: Third World Network and People's Health Movement, 2004, 23–6.

3. B Marston, KM de Cock. "Multivitamins, nutrition and antiretroviral therapy for HIV disease in Africa" (editorial). *New England Journal of Medicine* 351 (2004): 78–80.

4. SG Stolberg. "1997, Year of the crash: Despite new AIDS drugs, many still lose the battle." *New York Times*, 22 August 1997.

5. D Burton, RC Desrosiers, RW Doms, et al. "A sound rationale needed for phase III HIV-1 vaccine tests." *Science* 303 (16 January 2004).

6. R Belshe, G Franchini, MP Girard, et al. Letters. *Science* 305 (9 July 2004).

7. H Urnovitz. "On wasting even more public money on HIV vaccine trials." 7 July 2003. www.redflagsweekly.com/urnovitz/2003_jul07.html

8. J Cohen. "AIDS Vaccines: HIV dodges one-two punch." *Science* 305 (2004): 1545–7.

9. R Horton. "AIDS: The elusive vaccine." *New York Review of Books*, September 23, 2004. www.nybooks.com/articles/17400

10. HB Urnovitz. "AIDS: a 'host vs genome' disease with an associated 'virus.'" Statement for the Durban AIDS conference, 4 July 2000. www.chronicillnet.org/AIDS/durban.htm

11. KK Knox, DR Carrigan. "Disseminated active HHV-6 infections in patients with AIDS." *Lancet* 343 (1994): 577.

Index

Abrams, Dr. Donald, 50–51
acetaminophen, 100, 168–169, 192
Actuarial Association of South Africa, 1
Addy, Prof. P., 25
adrenal glands, 81, 138
  adrenocorticotropin hormone (ACTH), 81
AIDS (acquired immune deficiency syndrome)
causes of
    anti-AIDS drugs 18–19
    environmental toxins, 95, 126
    exhausted immune system, 110, 185, 187
    lifestyle, 17, 181
    polio vaccines, 88
    recreational drugs, 13, 15, 17, 19, 20, 73, 84, 90, 95, 147, 181
  chemotherapies, 9, 40, 159, 160, 162–63, 166, 181
  defined, 11, 16, 89
    Bangui definition, 5, 21
    lack of standardization, 180
  diagnosis, 5–6, 17
  exercise therapy, 174–178
    anti-VIP/NTM antibodies, 174, 176, 177, 178, 192
  in Uganda, 27–30, 34, 35, 57, 60, 72, 186, 187
  markers for, 7–9
    CD4 cell count, 6–8, 11–12, 17, 19, 37, 39, 41, 43, 46, 48, 50, 51, 74, 84, 85, 87, 93, 94, 95, 97, 98, 99, 105, 106, 113, 114, 115, 116, 117, 120, 121, 122–123, 125, 139, 146, 149, 154, 155, 161, 162, 163, 176, 178, 181
    HIV antibodies, 7, 17, 181, 189
    low levels of glutathione, 124
    oxidative imbalance, 124, 126
    viral load, 7, 12, 19, 24, 38, 39, 41, 74, 84, 85, 97, 113. 126, 149, 161, 162, 166, 181
  misdiagnosis, 22–23
  nutritional therapy for, 118–131, 193
  role of poverty, 17–18, 24, 100–101, 182
  treatment with generic drugs, 165–171

vaccines, 52, 53–75
  bacterial vector, 55
    Escherichia coli, 55, 57
    Listeria monocytogenes, 55
    Myobacterium bovis BCG, 55
    Salmonella, 55, 57
    Shigella, 55
    Streptococcus gordonii, 55
  death rates from, 64–65
  from plants, 60–61
  genetically engineered maize, 60, 65
  subunit, 54, 56
  trials of, 7–8, 42, 43, 53, 56, 57, 58, 60, 61, 63–75, 97, 98, 100, 183, 186, 187, 193
  viral vector, 55
    adenovirus, 55, 58, 64
    canarypox, 55, 59–60, 63, 72, 73
    fowlpox, 55, 72
    herpes simplex (HSV), 55, 58–59
    HIV-1 (rgp120), 55, 72–73
    HIV gp120/160, 66, 67, 74, 82, 84, 174–177, 185, 188, 192
    HIV/hepatitis B (HBV), 65
    HIV-SIV hybrid (SHIV), 64
    HSV-2, 58
    mutations in, 64, 66
    polio virus, 55
    V-1 Immunitor (V1), "the pink panacea," 74–75, 97–101, 165, 190
    vaccinia-gp160, 55, 59
    Venezuelan equine encephalitis (VEE), 55, 58, 72
    vesicular stomatis virus, 55
AIDS Conference in Durban, South Africa, 28, 89, 180, 182
  Durban Declaration, 15, 41, 180
AIDSmap, 71
AIDS Treatment News, 154
Albrecht, Dr. Carl, 148–149
alcoholism, 106
alfalfa mosaic virus, 60

About the Authors

Mae-Wan Ho

Dr. Mae-Wan Ho is director and co-founder of the Institute of Science in Society, London, U.K.; editor of *Science in Society*; scientific advisor to the Third World Network; and initiator and founding member of the Independent Science Panel. She is best known for her pioneering work on the physics of organisms and as a major critic of genetic engineering. Dr. Ho is a widely published author across many disciplines, and her books include *Genetic Engineering, Dream or Nightmare* (1998, 1999), *The Rainbow and the Worm, the Physics of Organisms* (1993, 1998, reprinted 1999, 2001, 2003); *Living with the Fluid Genome* (2003); and *GMO-Free: The Case for a Sustainable World* (2003, 2004).

Sam Burcher

Sam Burcher has a diploma in Art and Design from Camberwell School of Arts and Crafts and an ITEC Diploma in Anatomy and Physiology. She is able to combine her love of art and science as a researcher for the Institute of Science in Society (ISIS) and the Independent Science Panel (ISP). She also has a post-graduate diploma in Environment Education from London South Bank University and has campaigned for the environment for many years.

Rhea Gala

Rhea Gala has explored health issues from a variety of perspectives and has worked as an acupuncturist, as a counselor, and in conflict resolution. She has a first-class degree in Health and the Environment from the University of Wales and a Masters in Science degree in Biological Research Methods from the University of Exeter. Ms. Gala writes for the Institute of Science in Society on a variety of topics related to health and the environment. Like many people, she is greatly concerned for the future of the planet when those entrusted to protect it deny responsibility and evade accountability for their actions. Nevertheless, she believes in the power of community to transform us and reconnect us to our roots.

Veljko Veljković

Veljko Veljković earned his doctoral degree in Theoretical Physics from the Institute of Nuclear Science, Vinca, in 1973. He has conducted research and published numerous papers in this field, as well as in his other major areas of interest: Material Science, Biophysics, Bioinformatics, Protein Engineering, and AIDS Research. Currently working as an AIDS researcher at the Center of Multidisciplinary Research and Engineering at Vinca, Dr. Veljković has contributed considerably to the understanding of HIV, its protein envelope, and how the immune system recognizes or fails to recognize HIV by its protein signature. His current research is oriented toward the development of more effective AIDS therapy and prevention.

Check Out These Other Vital Health Titles!

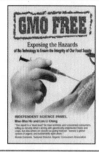
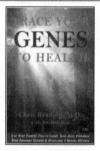
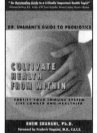
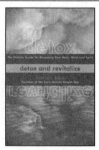